The Art School Dance

John Froy was born in Leeds in 1953 and grew up in south-west England. After taking a degree in Fine Art at Falmouth School of Art he taught English as a Foreign Language in London and Costa Rica for several years. Five months on an uninhabited island resulted in *On Cocos Island*, a fictionalised account and the start of his writing career, which was fuelled by further travels in Latin America. He settled in Reading in 1986 and set up a decorating business. Since then he has juggled decorating with writing: several unpublished novels, an account of his mother's death (*Mum, So Far*) and a volume of poetry *Eggshell: A Decorator's Notes*. In 2003 he took over Two Rivers Press which he co-ran for six years. He lives in Reading with his wife and daughter.

BY THE SAME AUTHOR

Eggshell: A Decorator's Notes (Two Rivers Press, 2007)
70 Waterloo Road: A childhood memoir 1953–1970 (Pine Wave Press, 2010)

ALSO PUBLISHED BY TWO RIVERS

All Change at Reading: the railway and the station: 1840–2013 by Adam Sowan
An Artist's Year in the Harris Garden by Jenny Halstead
The Ballad of Reading Gaol by Oscar Wilde
Believing in Reading: our places of worship by Adam Sowan
Birds, Blocks and Stamps by Robert Gillmor
Bizarre Berkshire by Duncan Mackay
Broad Street Chapel and the Origins of Dissent in Reading by Geoff Sawers
Charms against Jackals: 10 years of Two Rivers Press by Adam Stout and Geoff Sawers
Cloud Camera by Lesley Saunders
Down by the River: the Thames and Kennet in Reading by Gillian Clark
Eat Wild by Duncan Mackay
Eleven Rooms by Claire Dyer
Fair's Fair by Susan Utting
Foreigners, Drunks and Babies: eleven stories by Peter Robinson
From the Abbey to the Office: a short introduction to Reading and its writers by Dennis Butts
A Ladder for Mr Oscar Wilde by Geoff Sawers
A Mutual Friend: Poems for Charles Dickens edited by Peter Robinson
Newtown: a photographic journey in Reading 1974 by Terry Allsop
The Point of Inconvenience by A.F. Harrold
Reading poetry: an anthology edited by Peter Robinson
Scrimshaw by Jean Watkins
A Thames Bestiary by Peter Hay and Geoff Sawers

The Art School Dance

A memoir

John Froy

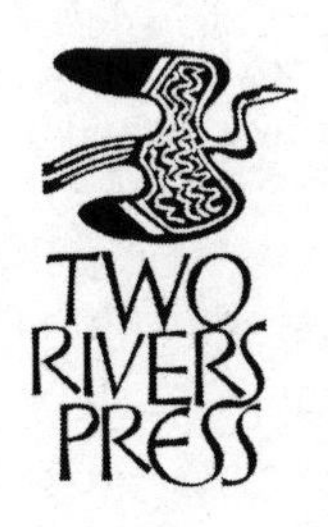

First published in the UK in 2013 by Two Rivers Press
7 Denmark Road, Reading RG1 5PA
www.tworiverspress.com

Copyright © Two Rivers Press 2013
Copyright © in text John Froy 2013
The author wishes to thank Giorgio Cipriani, Jane Farrell and Ray Atkins for their permission to reproduce the images on pp. 160 and 166

The right of John Froy to be identified as the author of the work has been asserted by him in accordance with the Copyright, Designs and Patents Act of 1988.

All rights reserved. No part of this publication may be reproduced, stored in or introduced into a retrieval system, or transmitted, in any form, or by any means (electronic, mechanical, photocopying, recording or otherwise) without the prior written permission of the publisher.

ISBN 978-1-901677-95-9

1 2 3 4 5 6 7 8 9

Two Rivers Press is represented in the UK by Inpress Ltd and distributed by Central Books.

Cover and text design by Nadja Guggi and typeset in Bembo and Parisine
Printed and bound in Great Britain by Imprint Digital, Exeter.

ACKNOWLEDGEMENTS
For all their help with the manuscript and nurturing of this book my special thanks to Elke Asmus, Clare Welsby, Jane Seraillier, Myra Cottingham, Paul Martin, Peter Robinson, David Grubb, the Stones Room Writers, Pagan Cruit, Mark Fry, Lisa Chaney, Edward Chaney, Ray Atkins, Deirdre Hyde and Naomi.

This is a true account as far as I remember. Some names have been changed in order to protect privacy.

Contents

Part Three: From Alba to Marrakesh

In memory of Lionel Miskin

'Things may come and things may go
but the art school dance goes on for ever'
— PETE BROWN

Part One: Italy, Reading and Colham

1. Painting in Porto Ercole

At last we've saved enough money to get to Italy. In February 1971 Lise and I hitch away from the English winter in Bedford, and head for Casa Fry, a villa at Porto Ercole, north of Rome. We take the train to Dover. Get off the ferry at Ostende and stick out our thumbs. The rucksack is stuffed with artists' materials as well as our clothes for two seasons. Lise's guitar has been left behind – a regret when we see how many hitchers with guitars there are along the roads of Europe. But we are seasoned hitchhikers after our great post-A-level trip to the south of Spain last summer; in England hitching has become the usual way of getting around. We make cardboard signs – FRANKFURT, MÜNCHEN, SALZBURG – stand by the road, expecting cars to stop, willing them to pull over.

When they don't, Lise goes out in front so the drivers see only her – it's normal practice, this courting with danger: boy hides in the ditch, girl gets the driver to stop; crazy. But in Belgium, Germany and Austria we don't need to resort to that. The lifts come easily, long fast rides down the autobahn. I don't think we even pause for the night, just carry on hitching. I remember feeling danger once, when a Turkish lorry draws up at 2 a.m. on the outskirts of Salzburg and we don't get in. We just wave him on. We'll wait. In Italy, on the outskirts of Bologna, a little white Fiat stops. We'll never fit into that! But the door opens and we squeeze in with our gear. Then it turns out the guy isn't going anywhere, he's playing some game. So we make him stop *now* and let us out. 'Pervert!' we yell as he moves away.

We reach Florence – Firenze – and find my friend Mark Fry, whose parents' house we are heading for in Porto Ercole. Mark is starting on a painting course at the Accademia di Belle Arti.

He gets us a crash pad, a patch of floor in the corridor of some rooms filled with American art students. He himself is staying at 'Laura's', an enormous apartment inside a *palazzo*. He puts on George Harrison's new triple LP, *All Things Must Pass*, and we lounge on the white leather sofas. Mark gets out his guitar. He's writing his own songs now. He sings us a new one about his new half-brother Wilde: 'March on my brother, go a little bit further.' It's a lovely song. There's a chance of making a record in Rome, he tells us, and jokes about Fry making it big.

Why don't we stay and do the painting course, though? He'll fix us up with somewhere to live. This is a genuine offer, I know, and persuasive. I know Mark. We were childhood best friends. In his garden at the age of four we pricked our fingers with a pin, mingled the blood in a saucer, rubbed it in, stinging, and became blood brothers. He would love us to stay, hang out in Florence with him. But this private painting course isn't my scene. Who would pay for it, anyway? I can't just 'get some lolly off my dad'. I've been to interviews for English art schools and if I get in, I'll apply for a local authority grant. Mark's world is diverging from mine – I touch his world, then glance off. Things aren't the same now I'm with Lise.

We linger in dizzying Florence, see the Uffizi and Pitti, the Duomo, the Donatello doors; Mantegna's solemn frescoes and the lighter, perfectly balanced Piero della Francescas; Michelangelo's stark naked *David* in a public square. Then we wander through the city without any plan, discovering little churches and piazzas for ourselves. Enter a nameless church, drawn in by the practising choir, sit and listen to spine-tingling Pergolesi; drift on, spend all day discovering, and arrive back to a glorious pink and orange postcard sunset on the Ponte Vecchio. With Mark and his friends we climb to Fiesole one day and picnic in a flower meadow as they did in E.M. Forster's *A Room with a View*. But we don't settle down, enticing though all this is. We were always going on to Porto Ercole.

So we hitch away down the Autostrada del Sole. In Orvieto, we admire the fabulous medieval cathedral façade and enter through bronze doors only made last year – though we don't know this, deliberately. We don't read up on a place, don't want to be told about it; we want to experience it fresh and first hand, be happily ignorant in our tourism, like those Forster characters eschewing their Baedekers. Lise is entranced by the hand-painted ceramics for sale in the cathedral square and we buy a small plate, stow it in the rucksack, hope it won't break. Then hitch on across country to Grosseto, Orbetello and Porto Ercole, walk up the long white dusty track to a house somewhere on the mountain.

I have a colour slide, blotchy with mould and fugitive colours, of a dark-haired girl in a long white old-fashioned nightdress, sitting outside at breakfast. The table is bright with Orvieto crockery. It's a sunny morning on the terrace at Casa Fry, the scrubby trees sprinkled with blossom, the valley below softly shadowed and dotted with olive groves and vineyards. All around lies the marvellous landscape I'm trying to paint.

'You must go,' Lise says.

But to which one?

We are still talking about the letter we picked up at the *poste restante* in the port. I have a place at Reading University to do History of Art with Fine Art in the autumn. This has come hot on the heels of an offer for Painting at Camberwell School of Art. Another lifeline. I know what I'm doing, there's a direction again.

'Maybe History of Art *and* Fine Art is the better option for you, Johnny.'

She's the only person who has ever called me that. Little parts of you, your name, can get claimed forever. In love, glowing, I fetch canvas and easel. Squeeze fresh oil colours on the palette, hold it in one hand, brushes in the other. I'm outdoors in the sun and breeze and insect-buzz, the spicy herb smells from the mountain. My first *plein air* painting on a modest rectangle of canvas board is on the easel.

The ever-shifting sun and shadows are a problem. The landscape won't stop still. How quickly the sun moves round, changing the shape of everything. And such a lot of it: slant of hill, silvery olive trees, vineyards, old fort on the skyline, distant block of sea, the high horizon. And what about the goats that come clonking through in the mornings? Shall I put them in too?

I remember my father talking about there being no lines in a landscape. 'Only shape and mass of colour,' he said, squinting down the Colham valley in Wiltshire where he lives and I still visit. 'On a two-dimensional surface, you have to abut your colours and tones. Lay them side by side. That's painting.'

In truth this was well over my head. I see lines everywhere. There are as many lines as there are tones and colours if you look for them. But what he picked on was my trying to put everything in as I sketched the view of the valley from his attic window; I didn't yet know what I wanted to select.

I take off my glasses and screw up my eyes, and at once the distracting detail merges, simplifies into blocks, shapes – there's some advantage in being short-sighted. The paint thickens up. I work at it, blend it; I'm getting used to the oil paint staying wet and malleable for days. But is it finished? I don't know. Every day the landscape is different, the mood changed. It has certainly given me trouble.

'How's it going? There's a bit of red.' Lise is still in her nightdress, barefoot on the stony ground. She probably won't get dressed until afternoon, or not at all if we aren't going anywhere.

'How are the studies going?' I counter.

'They're not. I've been reading. Whatever they say about Lawrence, he reads well out here. I like *Women in Love.*'

'So complicated. Like this painting. Give me *Sons and Lovers* any day. What red?'

'There.'

Much easier has been a pencil drawing of the same view, the olive groves and lines of vines each with their shadow – at least I knew when it was finished. I've been trying to draw Lise's portrait too, but can't get her likeness. Something my mother said about my father: 'Oh, he can paint but could never get a likeness.' She herself used to be an excellent portraitist. In her old portfolio at home there are many fine pencil portraits, as well as figures, nudes, cats, dogs, flowers.

'A lot of artists in your family, aren't there?' she says, hanging around. 'So this Granny Helen we're going to meet is another one!'

Besides my mother and father, my paternal grandmother Helen paints – though Dad says she's just a dabbler, she's really an actress. My stepfather Frank also paints. He's an art teacher and says he *only* dabbles, but he does a lot of it in his spare time. My sister Clare is thinking of doing a foundation course at Taunton Art School. And here I am doing the same.

'It's so good you've found something you really want to do, though. Because you hadn't only six months ago, when you left school.' She steals behind me and puts her arms round my neck as I squint at the landscape. Yes, all I wanted to do after school was travel and fall in love. Get away from home. I applied to university to read French at Norwich and then Sussex and didn't get in. It was only during the following winter the idea entered my head that I might want to do art after all. I gathered together my youthful work into a portfolio and took it for interview at Camberwell, and got a place. I took it to Reading – and now I've got in there, too.

'So when are you going to do your A levels, Lise?'

'Don't know.'

She never finished at Taunton Tech. It seems ridiculous that she hasn't taken a whole bunch of A levels and passed them with stars, she's so much brighter than me. But she hasn't, she keeps chopping and changing. I can well see the difficulty in getting down to them out here.

'We can go down to the port in a while.'

'Well, I'm not staying to clean the house!'

''Course you're not. Feminist.' For which I get a punch in the arm.

In fact we clean the little villa jointly without discussion. It's simple enough. One large room, two bedrooms behind it, a shower room between. No electricity, lighting by oil lamps, cooking on a small gas ring. Smells of garlic and oregano and damp from the shower. Scorpions in the crevices; we take a torch walking barefoot at night, check our shoes in the morning. The breakfast terrace is just outside the door. There are bay trees and cork trees, a large and wonderful olive tree, and now in the spring the mountain has a covering of wild flowers. It's a perfect little Lawrentian hideaway.

Though we aren't quite alone. Pat has the small bedroom. When we arrived we found the artist Patrick Symons was staying too, on his Easter vacation; Mark had said he might be. But Pat doesn't bother us, we hardly see him. He's out drawing all day and only comes home to sleep.

We set off for the port. Rather than use the long dusty track, we head straight down through the vineyards and olive groves – no matter that it's private land. I roughly know the way. The modern flat-roofed house we pass, and can see from our terrace, belongs to the writer Alan Moorehead.

'Met the Sainsburgers there once. You know *the* Sainsburys.'

'You don't have to name-drop to me, you know,' she says but she is impressed.

'We went to dinner as kids. Actually, what I really remember about that evening was Mark's sister, Lucy, singing 'Suzanne' a cappella, incredibly beautifully. First Leonard Cohen song I ever heard.'

I tell her about how Mark was friends with Alan Moorehead's son, Richard, who had a wonderful Pyrenean mountain dog; when I came here on holiday we made an expedition to the ruined sixteenth-century Spanish fort, climbed the great ramparts, entered the fort, with this great white dog leading us all the way. I have only a vague recollection of Alan Moorehead from that time, on the beach and going to see his adventurer friend Dick Waller who had accompanied him on his famous trip to the source of the Nile. On that last occasion, with the Sainsburys, he was already paralysed and almost dumb from his stroke. I didn't discover what a well-known travel writer and intrepid war correspondent he was until years later.

Down on the tarry fishy quay of Porto Ercole, Lise and I eat hot slivers of pizza in a slip of greaseproof paper. We buy wine, bread, cheese, pasta, tins of fish. The smell of roasted coffee beans is everywhere and irresistible. We splash out on espressos in a waterfront café. I add spoonfuls of sugar to the tiny cup, turning it almost into syrup.

I met Lise a year ago over a coffee in her family's café in my home town of Wellington in Somerset. The Coffee Shop had appeared, miraculously, on my route to school. It was run by a plump Australian woman and her beautiful daughters, Anna and Lise, and it drew me in like a magnet. They were a talkative lot, especially the mother. No, they were all equally talkative, including the brainy younger brother, and nothing at all like my family. I stayed for hours in their shop over a single cup of coffee. I soon fell in love with Lise. I fell so deeply in love with her I didn't dare tell her. I talked and talked and waited. I waited five months, until I'd done my A levels, then hitched off to Spain with her.

When we got back, I left home with her. I joined Lise and her sister Anna in their first flat in Bristol. No one in the flat had a job. Anna was looking for work, she was actually after a real job in a children's home, but Lise and I weren't even trying; we were just interested in living away from home. We scrimped through the autumn of 1970 on the dole, kept a fire going in the coal grate, burning scrap wood gleaned from the local shops and building sites. We stayed up most of the night, still talking, and working out the chords of *Abbey Road* on the guitar; we made pancakes at midnight, toast and jam at dawn, went for walks on Redlands Downs in the first light.

Then we all went home at Christmas. In the New Year we tried again, another flat, in Bedford this time with Anna's boyfriend, Paul, who was at college there. We were a household of two young couples now; I was still only seventeen, Lise had just turned eighteen. I got a job in the new Cranfield Institute, a few miles out of the town. This was by some margin the best job I'd had – potentially a real job – and I hoodwinked the Director to get it. I felt bad about that. He took me on in good faith, believing I really would start from the bottom, the old way, a school-leaver with promise, and rise up through the ranks. He said he would be able to help with college training later. He presented his job with such charm: if I stayed under the protecting and cherishing arm of the Institute, he said, I could go up and up, the world my oyster.

But I wasn't charmed, I wasn't thinking that way at all. I saw the clerical work was dull as ditchwater and knew I wouldn't stay long. Just long enough to save up some cash. Lise meanwhile was a silver service waitress in Bedford. She too had bluffed her way in, even more than I had – how could you learn silver service if no one would take you on and train you in the first place? Of course she said she was experienced and of course we'd seen *Catch-22*.

We went to the movies that winter in Bedford. Bergman's *The Touch*, Visconti's *Death in Venice*, Zeffirelli's *Romeo and Juliet*, the film of D.H. Lawrence's *The Virgin and the Gypsy*. It was classy cinema with Lise – no more 007 and spaghetti westerns for me for a while. But it was also beautiful cinema, serious, intensely romantic; it was the discovery of great European cinema.

And in the evenings I drew. I started copying Van Gogh drawings from a great monograph my mother had given me for my seventeenth birthday (it had cost her an arm and a leg). Mum loved Van Gogh, and, I was discovering, so did I. I started with his early *Potato Eaters*, drew his workingman's boots in thick charcoal. Drew my own suede desert boots in the same manner, rubbing and smearing the paper with my fingers. And pollarded willows beside dykes and canals, which looked like the flat Bedfordshire landscape the minibus drove through on its way to Cranfield.

Van Gogh's story was exciting too. Our longing to go south to the Mediterranean in part mirrored Vincent's escape from Paris to Provence when the almond blossom was out. When I told Lise about my friend Mark's house in Italy, she immediately wanted to go there. She seemed like an Italian herself, the way she gesticulated when she spoke, her intensity; she insisted her name was Li*s*a, pronounced the Italian way, though I still called her Li*z*e. Yes, I was sure we'd be able to live in Porto Ercole for a while. We made plans: we would hitch out there, live simply. I would paint the Italian landscape; she would work on her A levels, read, learn Italian. We trekked down to Box in Wiltshire to see Mark and his father Tony (another artist). It was as I thought. 'Sure, stay as long as you want,' Tony said in his super-relaxed way. 'Super girl,' he whispered when Lise was out of the room.

She was, she was such a lovely girl, and I could still hardly believe I was living with her.

The provisions from the port are lugged back up the hill. We find a wild tortoise in the grass – it lumbers away – then almost tread on a black and yellow viper warming itself in the sun. Landscape painters, out in the scrub all day, quiet for hours, should remember snakes come out when it's quiet.

'Wonder if Pat'll be in for supper tonight,' Lise says.

'He really doesn't want us to worry about him.'

'He was nice about the marmalade.'

Pat shared his marmalade with us on our first morning. The only thing he couldn't live without when abroad, he laughed. A friend of my father's, he had appeared from time to time during my childhood; he was an expert botanist as well as a painter, knew the names of all the wild flowers on a walk.

'We've hardly seen him.' She sounds disappointed. Lise is more interested in people than me. I don't think I'm very interested in people at all. 'He's homosexual, isn't he?' she says.

'Is he?'

I haven't realised in all this time. It was never mentioned at home. *That's* it. The indefinable little difference. The curious stare he sometimes pinned you with. I know next to nothing about homosexuality – it's still very much closet. We don't use the word 'gay' yet.

I've discovered a simple rule of outdoor painting: work at the same time each day for about two hours, until the sun moves round and the light changes the shape of everything. I like my steeply angled hill, a strong diagonal, which I can balance with the sea horizon and distant fort. By keeping squinting, I don't get too much detail in. I see the mass of things. But the colour is difficult, as always. I started with a grey sky because it was grey that day, and I've kept it grey, though the sun is out now. I like grey with the yellows of last year's grasses, the fresh spring green of the bushes and the silvery olives.

Indoors, I sketch a vase of flowers in brown ink, which reminds me of my mother's ink drawing. Monochrome is easy. Then I do a bright still life of the Orvieto ceramics clustered on the table in oil pastels, dipping my finger in turps to soften and meld the colours – like a Bonnard postcard Mum sent me. Lise reads in the wicker chair. There are orange D.H. Lawrence Penguins are scattered round the house. We read scenes from *Lady Chatterley* together aloud, shock ourselves with the Anglo-Saxon words: 'Th'art good cunt, though …' says Mellor. 'What is cunt?' says Connie … 'It's like fuck, then?' 'Nay, nay! Fuck's only what you do. Animals fuck. But cunt's a lot more than that.' We celebrate my eighteenth birthday in the little house on the Italian hill. At dusk, light the oil lamps at dusk, cook up our *spaghetti napolitana*, drink some wine, play Hangman and Consequences, and go to bed.

'Hares and rabbits,' says Lise as soon as she wakes.

'Pinch and a punch for the first of the month,' I counter.

We take this little superstition quite seriously. Just as we have faith in the Stars: my Arian 'fire', her Scorpion 'sting'. The atypical side of my Arian nature – not pushy, soft – is tempered by my mother's Sagittarian aspect, apparently, according to some mysterious Zodiac calculations we have made.

Pat is going back to England. He shows us some 'very black' drawings of bee orchids, feigns horror and disgust at the plethora of grubby pencil marks he has made on the paper, laughing uproariously. He drives off down the track and that's the last time I ever see him. A few years later, I'll find his work in a Royal Academy Summer Show – those very same bee orchids, as well as a large Porto Ercole landscape done from further up the mountain. Then, years after that, I hear, he was with a group of art students in Paris and crossed the road looking the wrong way. Poor Patrick Symons was actually hit and killed by a bus.

We set off hitching to the south of Italy. Hitching requires no planning. Pack the rucksack, walk down the track in the early morning and stick out a thumb. It's a joy being on the road again in the May sun. We inch and jump our way down to Rome. I don't think we stay in Rome, oddly. We're soon in Naples and don't linger there either; the air around the station feels so thick with danger, with pickpockets, we're sure to lose everything within hours. So we take a local train out to Pompeii. Better to wander freely round these grassy ruins, pick up fragments of mosaic from a Roman rubbish dump. Better to stay in a monastery.

Having moved a little further south and arriving randomly, as you do when hitching, we need somewhere to stay that evening and decide to try a monastery. Lise is confident the monks will take us in. We climb a dusty road on the edge of town of Buccino, knock on the great door of the Franciscan monastery there. A small door within the door opens and we are welcomed inside. In a flurry of activity, two folding beds are set up in a large room, we are brought a small table and chairs and some supper. Our breakfast is brought for us in the morning. A novice monk, Alain, who speaks some English, gives us a tour of the monastery; we pose outside with him and a priest for a photograph. Their hospitality has been overwhelming.

We go only a little further. Stuck on a mountain road on the way to Potenza, we ask: Why are we always trying to hitch through to somewhere else? Why are we always on the road? We should take hold of this wonderful wooded landscape around us, be here now. So we leave the road for a while and climb down into the deep valley, take off shoes and pick our way across the river. An old man shows us his hut built of grass and reeds and says we can rest there. We stay in his hut by the water through the heat of the day, eat what food we have. Leaving the hut, I throw Lise's shoes across the river and one falls short. She's furious, unjustly, it seems to me; the shoe is soaked but not ruined. 'Arian!' she accuses. 'Scorpion!' I defend. We climb back to the road and cross over, start hitching the other way, back to Porto Ercole. Sitting with our thumbs out on the quiet stretch of mountain road, Lise says, 'Let's write about the landscape, if we can't draw it.' So we both write a descriptive piece on what we can see from the road, our experience at the river. Her writing is fresh, different; she always chooses the right word.

Our stay at Porto Ercole comes to an end. That's to say, the money finally runs out. We set off for England with my new portfolio of artwork, following the coast road this time, through Pisa and Genoa and into France. Our ride down the switchbacks into Monaco is actually with a racing driver, who is only too keen to demonstrate; it all seems like part of a movie as we come screeching down into this playground of the rich. Our rally driver drops us and somehow we manage to go off with his ID card. Lise will find it at home weeks later and send it to him: 'Hope you aren't in prison!'

Hitching along the Côte d'Azur is easy. We walk though Nice, past whispered offers of hashish from Algerians along the waterfront, and head on to Antibes to call on Granny Helen. She lives in the village of Biot and has no idea we are coming. Nor have I ever been there. I hardly know my exotic Granny who lives in Provence, who is a painter now and used to be an actress, have only ever seen her twice before when I was a child. I call from a kiosk in Antibes. It's all a bit Graham Greeneish – indeed the mysterious Greene was living in Antibes at the time; that rare clip of him striding along the quay was filmed here. And the Rolling Stones, tax-exiles, were making their *Exile on Main Street* record at Nellcôte, a few miles away.

Granny Helen appears unfazed by my call. 'Stay where you are and I'll pick you up,' she says briskly. We turn up at her doorstep and she takes us in. I meet Tully, her second husband, with whom she has built her second or third life in the South of France. They settled here in the late fifties, at first in the old *Four*, an ex-bakery, then moved to a modern villa at the edge of the village. We have dinner on the terrace, where they eat almost all the year round, so mild are the winters. They can't stand the lingering cold in England.

'Oh nor can I,' Lise, child of Australia and Fiji, agrees.

'Miserable,' says Helen.

'Absolutely,' Tully concurs.

'This melon's *piquant*, wouldn't you say?'

'*Piquant*,' echoes Tully.

'These paintings … are they real?' Lise says. It's what we've both been thinking.

They laugh. Helen and Tully get on so well. And it's evident from the start that Helen will get on with Lise. Yes, the paintings are originals. The walls are covered with works of art. Incredibly, the large oil over the mantelpiece in the sitting room is by Paul Delvaux. Its moonlit scene of figures in a ruin is both romantic and erotic; the women are very naked with their bushes of pubic hair. There's an Edward Bawden which will end up in the Tate. In the hall by the phone, a small Picasso ink drawing. Pablo, the local lad just over the hill at Mougins, Granny Helen jokes, shrewd, beady-eyed. Indeed Helen, who has always been said to have 'a good eye', has invested substantially in art. She bought Francis Bacon when he was unknown and keeps them in a bank vault in Paris; they will pay for healthcare in her and Tully's old age.

But my grandma is a bundle of health and energy now. Having shown us round her little house with its amazing art on the walls, she takes us up to the *Four*, now her studio, where we will sleep. I don't recall seeing any of her own artwork here – perhaps it was turned to the wall – instead, she tells us about the famous local pottery and the Fernand Léger Museum in Léger's house. It's a serendipitous and joyful stay in Biot. We sleep at the *Four*, look round the pretty pottery-filled village. Helen cooks delicious meals. She takes us to the beach at Antibes, where she and Tully swim every morning at eight. They dip in the briny Med, do the required number of strokes, are out and gone in fifteen minutes. Lise and I stay on the beach and catch the bus back for another of Helen's tasty lunches – such a treat after life on the road. Her two tabby cats have it good too, tucking into their chopped fillet steak, 'only the best'. One is called Raoul and he raouls for his supper.

Helen and Tully enjoy good conversation with the meal and after our travels in Italy we feel we can supply some of that. Granny Helen tells us interesting things too. She trained at RADA and played Sorrel Bliss in Noel Coward's *Hay Fever* in 1925; she co-starred with Laurence Olivier in *The Rats of Norway* in 1933. She happily talks about her acting career but doesn't mention her divorce, my father and his brother being sent off to boarding school at a very young age, nor anything of her three children with Tully, with the exotic names of Pagan, Lyn and Hippolyte, my step aunt and uncles whom our side of the family have never met. At home Mum once showed me a newspaper cutting of Aunt Pagan, *Vogue* model. Our Granny Betty, her mother, was always scouring the *Express* for articles and she found this one on Pagan before she went off to Los Angeles. I'd like to know more about these unknown relatives but it seems that Helen like my father prefers to steer clear of 'family'.

Still, the Granny Helen of here and now is good enough for me. She's even been to a Joan Baez concert 'out in the hills with the hippies'. She *likes* hippies, their colourful clothes and attitude, their optimism and message of peace.

'Please call me Helen,' she says. 'Granny makes me feel old.'

The moment has come to show my portfolio.

'This interest in art is quite new. I don't remember you having it before.'

It's true I didn't take art at school – only the academic subjects; I did German instead of art. But I painted and drew at home on my own. Mostly fairly standard teenage fare – fantasy and the fantastic, inspired by my love of Tolkien – but there were also attempts at rendering the landscape as the eye sees it. I was interested in the real landscapes behind the dwarves and dragons.

Helen is looking through with some interest. She gets to the end, threads her way back, and pronounces the work 'has something'. She picks out a quick pen and ink sketch. She likes a pencil drawing 'with a touch of Cézanne'. My *pièce de résistance*, the oil painting of the hillside, is less successful. 'Doesn't quite come off.'

'It's the colour,' I say.

'Of course colour is *the* most difficult thing in painting,' Helen says.

But she praises the portfolio, is pleased I'm going to art school, which is a fine feather for my cap. Praise from Helen is praise indeed.

We aren't allowed to carry on hitching. Sweetly, Helen and Tully buy us boat-train tickets to Victoria and take us to the station. Helen makes us promise to come and see her when she's next in London.

2. Two homes

We go home to Somerset. Wellington is smaller after nine months away. I'm back in my mother's house at Waterloo Road, with Lise up the road at her mother's coffee shop. Strangely, we've suddenly stopped living together. After Bristol, Bedford and Italy we are now 'going out' again. Home with my mum and stepfather Frank and sisters all seems very strange and cramped.

Lise and I both come from broken homes. Of course this hasn't affected *us*, we say, it's pretty normal, happens to many people we know. Nevertheless our parents', well, our dads', behaviour, greatly interests us. Lise's father left home when she was in her early teens. My father earlier on, when I was four or five. Hers settled in a new relationship. Mine didn't for years, he was all over the place right through the sixties. Her mother hasn't remarried – Lise describes their exodus from London, how they, her mother, two sisters and brother, came down to live in Devon and then Somerset almost as fugitives. My mother married Frank in 1960. My sisters and I, split up at the time of the divorce, were reunited at Frank's house in Wellington and it became our home.

My sisters are Clare, Catherine and Sarah. Sarah is my half-sister, Frank and my mother's daughter, born three years after we all came back together. Clare is sixteen, and now definitely leaving grammar school in Taunton to go to the art school next year. Catherine is thirteen and at the local comprehensive. Sarah is seven and at the primary school C and C went to. I went to boarding school when I was seven and missed my sisters' early school years, only seeing them in the holidays. I wasn't around when Sarah was born (mother and baby were still in hospital the day of Kennedy's assassination). I've only known my sisters since I was thirteen and came home to go to Wellington School up the road, where Frank teaches.

Frank takes us upstairs to Clare's bedroom for the photos. It's currently also home to her two blue budgies, Fili and Kili, and the door has to be kept closed at all times because of the cat. The room receives good north light from a large window and the 'portrait chair' is beside the window; sometimes there's a white umbrella set up above it to reflect extra light downwards. Here Frank takes his portraits of the family growing up and his special portraits of Mum-looking-beautiful in a new outfit or hat.

'Just a couple for the album if you can bear it?' he says. 'Otherwise there'll be a gap.' He fixes his old Rolleicord camera to the tripod.

Lise and I stand together behind the chair. With our Italian tans we look well.

It's still only June, a long time until September. I get a job at the local chrysanthemum nursery. Lise is helping her mother in the coffee shop; she'll be doing her A levels by correspondence now, as she doesn't know where she will be next.

I cycle out to Rockwell Green and am inducted into the adult day of eight hours of physical work, which seems to me to be pure slave labour. I'm a disbudder. Chrysanthemums naturally branch all the way up the main stem, but that isn't what's wanted. The side shoots have be picked off, every one, repeatedly, to ensure a single large bloom per plant. I spend all day doing this, picking off thousands of little shoots, staining my fingers green with the pungent sap. Now the disbuddings are cuttings to be planted up in the greenhouse in their thousands, so at least they are used. Cuttings are preferable to disbudding but the place is still a factory churning out flowers.

Some of the flowers are strangely coloured. I ask the owner about this, the peculiar 'metallic' hues in the show greenhouses. He says it's the radiation. Yes, they've had a dose of radiation, the owner crows excitedly. They regularly send off flowers for 'treatment' at Hinkley Point, our local nuclear power station on the North Somerset coast, to get new colours, 'and you never know what you'll get back.'

'Get back to your work, you gert buggers,' yells the tyrant foreman riding around on his tractor. The work is shockingly hard, the hours long, the wages abysmal, but we slaves humbly obey. Sackings are common, on the slightest pretext. Apparently there are always people eager to replace us.

'What's this sludge?' I ask Gert Bugger about a mysterious brown heap in one of the greenhouses. Ingratiating of me, perhaps, but we've been told to steer clear of it. 'Someone said it was nicotine.' It *is* nicotine. Plant poison. They use it as a pesticide.

The odd extra-marital situation with Lise continues. We are still 'going out'. As far as her mother is concerned we don't sleep together, though we've been living with each other for the past nine months. This state of denial will persist for the rest of our relationship and cause all sorts of manoeuvring. We bypass it of course, as with any unreasonable request or instruction from a parent. We find time for each other when we can. There are occasions when her house is empty. My house always seems to be full of Mum and sisters, so we go down to the sports fields by the park and lie in the long grass like teenagers – like the teenagers we still are.

Then Lise misses a period and has a pregnancy scare, and we're discussing abortions, jolted out of our dreamy, haphazard lives. There's no question of us having the child, surely ... There always is, though, isn't there? There are always doubts, hopes ... No, she isn't going to tell her mother; she must get on and have the abortion right away. She makes an appointment with a gynaecologist, remotely in Taunton. 'Why are all gynaecologists male?' she complains afterwards. Then it goes away. Suddenly she isn't pregnant any more. It was either a phantom pregnancy or an early miscarriage. She won't miss her Pill in the future.

In the garden at home I draw the Albertine rose entwined in the trellis, the lovely pale pink flowers against dark glossy leaves. Frank planted it for Mum, one of her favourite roses, beautifully scented. He takes some of his outdoor family portraits by the Albertine. Lise and I talk about feminism, the new feminism, by the Albertine. Lise has been reading *The Female Eunuch.* She's isn't a feminist, she says, at least not the bra-burning sort. No, she's feminine. My difficulty with women's lib is that I already believe women are superior to men. They're gentler, kinder, more peaceful and understanding. They talk more. They're better. With enormous naïveté, I think they already have equal rights with men. It hasn't occurred to me that women are treated unfairly, badly, appallingly, as inferiors in the world of men. I find the whole underwear-burning business a bit weird.

And I don't know how any of this applies to my mother. Women's lib hasn't really entered our household, it isn't relevant. Mum doesn't go out to work because she 'can't'. She has never worked (apart from a year as teacher assistant in Carlisle during the war); she isn't qualified, has no training. She isn't really *well enough* to go to work. She stays at home and listens to Housewives' Choice. However, although she's a housewife, or 'house mum', she calls herself, she doesn't actually do any housework either. She starts but never finishes. We have to finish everything for her.

But she does praise my small square drawing of the rose and trellis, and I trust her on this. The drawing is a modest, slight thing, yet I will take it to Reading and base my first term's work on it. And she was complimentary about the little portfolio I brought back from Italy. Like Helen she's happy I'm going to art school, as she did. She says she likes my quick ink drawings best for their 'freshness', and looking afresh at *her* ink drawing of wild grasses in the sitting room, I can see new similarities, and how very much better it is than mine.

Of course she knows about my partial colour blindness, my *deficiency*. When I was drawing the Albertine rose, I could see the pink flowers against the dark green leaves. At least I thought I could. I can see them in my mind's eye now. I see many colours. But some of them are questionable. There are some unknown colours in the garden. Are the cranesbills more blue or purple? Are they lavender or mauve? The vermilion geraniums seem to vanish at a distance … Naturally, I've known this for years, ever since I famously uttered as a young child that a green double-decker bus in Bath was red like a London one and shocked my painter father. I've always missed things: the poppies in a cornfield that everyone admires from the car, 'a good year for holly berries', the wash of red on a roach's back in the canal at Bath, the pinkness of Devon earth. 'Ah, the pink country!' my father would cry as he drove us home to Wellington after our childhood holidays. But it hasn't been a problem so far. It has only prevented me from being a train engine driver or the captain of a ship. No, I see what I see. I just see differently from others. I have this disability. I'm putting myself into the lion's den by going to art school.

It's the school summer holidays and I go with my sisters to our father's. That's to say, with Clare and Catherine, as Sarah doesn't come – she never did come, it was always a source of tension in the holidays, when we went away and she stayed at home. It would have been helpful if she'd come along too, a healing and unifying thing for the family. Colham farmhouse is at Castle Combe in Wiltshire, by a river in its own valley, and idyllic. We've been having great holidays there with our dad since 1964. Swimming in the reedy By Brook, mucking about with a raft and tractor inner tubes, flymowing the rank grass, washing the car, digging the veg patch, walking, bird- and butterfly- and flower-spotting, collecting feathers as pipe cleaners for our dad; then tobogganing, wood-chopping and blazing log fires in the winter. We light a fire in summer too, when the August nights draw in with a nip in the air.

We don't know our artist father well. He lives another, invisible life. We only see him here in this house for the fun and games of holidays. We've only ever glimpsed our other dad – our real artist dad – through his studio door, the large room on the first floor, the best room in the house. He doesn't tell us but things are let slip, big things they seem to us: he did a mural, a mosaic, in the Belgrade Theatre, Coventry when it was rebuilt after the war; there's a newspaper cutting at home of a review of his most recent exhibition at the Hanover Gallery in 1968; he even put in for the Sydney Opera House competition in 1957, he said, with 'a very trad square design'. And of course he teaches painting at Chelsea School of Art. That's to say, as our mother would say with blatant envy, he actually lived and worked on the King's Road in the 60s.

Lise is invited to join us at Colham. The problem of co-habiting doesn't arise here. We're accepted by my dad and new stepmother, Catherine H, as a couple and even honoured with the new guest room in the attic. This of course is the very room we used the previous October on our Goldilocks weekend, our first frolic in the hay if you like, when I secretly brought my new girlfriend to my father's wonderful house and unknowingly we slept in his bed – he was less bothered by this than the impertinence of my 'breaking in' uninvited. But all has been forgiven. Lise has been to Colham legally since and gets on all right with my father and Catherine H, and now, perhaps to fully welcome her into the family, we've been given the double bed. I can still feel a lingering pride in this. The small 'green' room of my childhood and adolescence on the other side of the attic was now truly outgrown.

Lise loves Colham. We walk around the extent of it, the valley up to Castle Combe village and beyond to the source of the By Brook; the neighbouring valley, deep-cut, with no roads and a special quietness; then up the other side to Truckle Hill barn, site of a Roman villa, where we search the ploughed field for pottery shards or even a coin; and then down the valley, following the river to Long Dean, where the Hodgkins live. Julia Hodgkin enthused about my doing art history and has lent me Gombrich's *The Story of Art* as the best introduction to the subject. Their house, another mill on the By Brook like Colham, is filled with amazing Indian paintings collected by Howard. His paintings are all in his studio, which I've never seen inside; I remember once a fluent pencil sketch of one of their sons just propped against a wall – 'by David' (Hockney). We look at the house from the lane, then branch off up the rabbit valley, a favourite walk as a child, which had countless rabbits before myxomatosis came.

And she loves the beautiful old Colham house my father has done up, is still doing up, so simply, so elementally, with its white walls, oak beams and dark polished floors. It has a rough 'vernacular' feel: immensely thick walls that angle and curve, deep windowsills, a spiral wooden staircase, stone flags in the kitchen and 'dairy' outhouse; the woodshed with its bare stone walls where I'm helping my dad knock a way through to the garden.

But Lise doesn't get the silence of the meals. I suppose we don't notice it. Eating at my father's has always been a silent business; loud the clatter of cutlery on plates but few and far between the words; a kind of hushed reverence. For Lise this is far from any mealtime in her family, where you'd never stop anyone from talking.

'What's all the hush *for*?' she whispers.

I think of *The Virgin and the Gypsy* where the stultifyingly silent meals helped drive the virgin into the gypsy's arms. I think about my father's father, Grandpa William Alan Froy, 'WAF', and though I haven't had a meal at WAF's house since I was very young, I remember the awful posh silence of his dining table. WAF's silence has been inherited by his son. Granny Helen certainly never liked silence, which is maybe why she left WAF for Tully. Whereas her good cooking has passed down to her son. Colham is very much about Dad's great home cooking with homegrown veg from a bountiful garden. Meals there are silent but delicious, a combination of my father's parents.

My father is more circumspect about my portfolio than Mum or Helen. He knows of course that I'm going to Reading, and we have talked about it to some extent, but he has maintained an air of bemusement that I should want to do the same as he did. He says he doesn't want to encourage me on to such an uncertain path if I'm not really sure, which I almost take to be a Don't. He puffs away on his pipe, strokes his chin, looking through the portfolio. Father and mother and stepfather and grandmother *are* rather a lot of artists for one family, he raises his right eyebrow quizzically. Yes, he's most careful not to encourage me into a life in art, but then he doesn't encourage me in any other direction either.

Upstairs in the beautiful white bedroom with its oak beam and white counterpane, Lise says, 'He's rather lukewarm about you doing art. Is it the colour thing?'

'Oh, he's just being cautious. It's true I didn't do art at school. And I was going to university to do French only a year ago.'

'Not much help, though. Your family's strange,' she says.

'So's yours, all talking with their mouths full at meals.'

'And he's never even been to his mother's. Has she seen this beautiful house?'

'Only once, I think, one Easter holidays when I was here. It was the time she told me I was sexually frustrated for biting my nails! Dad cooked her favourite roast lamb. She brought him a special bottle of duty-free whisky he treasured.'

'But no return invitation?'

'It all goes back to the ban, you see. Sometime after the war, long after WAF and Helen had split up, Tully put this ban on her children from her previous marriage from ever visiting. I think it was when they had their chicken farm at Uckfield in Sussex. And the ban held. It's still holding now as far as I know. So Dad's never got to see his mum in Biot. And I've never met Tully's children.'

'Very strange,' she says.

My father, always reticent on matters of family history, opened up a little in his old age. Recently, he told me something of when he and my mother were together, one of the only things he has told me about 'Mum and Dad'. They were living in London and had been invited to Pagan's wedding. It was a grand do in Sussex, all paid for by *Vogue*. 'The whole thing was like a film set, a grand tableau.' But they missed it. 'Your mum was worked up and unwell at the time' and she made them so late they missed the ceremony. *His* mother never forgave him for that.

Back home in Waterloo Road, Frank has organised my grant application. It's always Frank who does this side of things. As I've said, Mum doesn't concern herself over any of the running of the house and our everyday needs. I don't suppose she could, but the fact remains I've grow up in a wholly male-run, Frank-run, household. Frank does the shopping, cooking, washing, vacuuming and ironing. We all do the washing up. Clare and Catherine do some of the washing and ironing now. The application form we sent off works out very well: I qualify for a full local authority grant based on my mother's income – which is zero! One bonus to having divorced parents, I suppose. In preparation for my art history I read *The Story of Art*. Lise and I aren't splitting up but she isn't coming with me to university.

3. Reading Fine Art

Paul gives me a lift up to Reading in his van. He's on his way from his home in Tiverton to Bedford, where he has a new flat for the autumn. Anna and Lise will be joining him there. Big bearded Paul, at ease, confident in the world, it always seems to me, drops me off at Child's Hall. I'm suddenly very small and alone in my box of a room.

My room overlooks the lake on the university's park-like campus. I go to lie on the grass by the lake. There are swans, ducks, and a bird I believe to be a great crested grebe, my first; there are no great crested grebes in south-west England at the time, they are still making their comeback from their slaughter by the Victorian hat industry. It turns out these most elegant aquatic birds are resident on Whiteknights Lake right on my doorstep and I can see them every day. Everyone feels alone, don't they? Many are leaving home for the first time. My loneliness is both for leaving home – again – and for being separated from Lise. It must also contain shades of my termly dumping at boarding school from the age of six to thirteen.

Back indoors the corridors are smelling strongly of food. The evening meal is a stuff-up of meat, vegetables and pudding; I join other freshers going to the disco in the girls' hall, Bridges, across the lake. It seems so silly. I already have my girl, I've been living with her for a year. I stand at the side and drink a lot of beer, meet a guy who's reading the new subject of Cybernetics.

It's the tail end of the week and courses don't start until Monday. Things take a long time to get going for us freshers. Very laid back, you could say, but also an alarming stretch of unstructured time. I register in the morning, Friday morning, and that only takes an hour. I look round the Students' Union, see a lot of political posters – 'agitprop' – learn there's a sit-in at the Faculty of Letters. I pass the banners on my way to the library with my booklist for the year: History of Art, Sociology and Anthropology. The Department of Fine Art isn't on the main campus but half a mile away down on London Road.

I meet De Gruyter in the Union. He's already found someone else on the Fine Art course, and we sit and have tea in the cafeteria. De Gruyter has Paul's self-confidence in even larger quantities. He has come to do a combined Fine Art with History of Art degree like me. Airily and extraordinarily he speaks critically of our course before we've even started it. He seems to know quite a bit about the staff already, is almost hostile before we meet them. He presents me with the names of his heroes Wyndham Lewis and the Vorticists, whom I've never heard of, and proceeds to lay into 'modern art'. I don't know what to say; I compare Helen's approach to art; I compare my father's opinions, which, though secretive and understated, are certainly modern. But De Gruyter seems to latch on to me right from the start and I'm grateful for the support. I happily tuck under his wing.

Down at the studios on Monday morning, De Gruyter sets up impressively with a large half-completed portrait of T.S. Eliot on his easel. I choose my studio space nearby, get myself a 'donkey' and drawing board. The room is full of expectant faces. We sit astride our donkeys and listen to the course tutor Alan Plummer talk on. I wonder now what he said and what we did for our first exercise. Large sheets of cartridge paper and work freely? Something unfettered with cardboard boxes? From his corner De Gruyter mocks our tutor's 'trendy' sheepskin jerkin and jeans; what the man's saying is all too open-ended and woolly for him. But Reading Fine Art is modern, progressive, very much concerned with the Art of Now. Rita Donagh did her *White Room* experiments here in 1970, where the model in a life-drawing class melds into the group drawing her in a white room. Subtle and poetic abstract artist Prunella Clough has been a visiting tutor. Installation artists Richard Wilson and Cornelia Parker will come here.

I need to make a start of my own. The work from Porto Ercole isn't going to be of much use here. I get out my drawing of the Albertine rose and trellis and expand it to A1 size. It's about 'looking through' a lattice of forms to the garden beyond. I work in acrylics, and for now stick safely to monochrome, drawing with the paint. Something promising does appear but I'm unsure how to carry on with it. No one comes to advise me. I feel so far removed from the original subject here – I don't know how to work away from the subject. Seeking fresh inspiration, I decamp to the Soil Science greenhouses, which are somewhat incongruously attached to Fine Art and more exotic than they might sound with their ornate cream-painted cast ironwork and cascading plants. I spend some time sketching in there. Someone called Jane, whom I hardly knew on the course and haven't seen since, recently sent a photograph of me with my corkscrew hair seated there, sketchbook on knee. But no one minds me working there, or anywhere, provided I bring in something to show them. My tutor, Harry Redmond, a printmaker, is easygoing: it seems I can do as I like so long as I do something.

In my men's hall I stuff myself with the stodgy food three times a day, making the most of these paid-for meals. I sit with the guy from Cybernetics. Girls, sport and rock music are the topics of conversation. I have my girl – she's living in Bedford – and sport isn't anywhere on my radar. The Who are playing at the Students Union – am I going with Cybernetics and the others? My musical interests are now tending to follow Lise's: Bach, Beethoven, Scarlatti, Couperin; as with literature and film, I've been going through a steady induction into the classical greats. But I did go to a stunning Who concert at the Bristol Hippodrome in my last year at school, when they played their rock opera *Tommy*, and I wouldn't mind ... I dither, then the concert is sold out anyway.

I miss Lise badly. She writes, saying how she misses me. She's bought a blue velvet dress from the Oxfam in Bedford 'for only two shillings', which she thinks I'll get cross about. We've always had so little money, Lise and I; the months it took us to rake together enough to buy her new guitar strings. She is studying hard for her A levels in the town library and doing embroidery in the evenings – how that surprises me now but there it is in the letter, one of the saved love letters still in their pale blue Basildon Bond envelopes with a new decimal 3p stamp.

I investigate the sit-in at the banner-draped Faculty of Letters. It's three years since '68, the LSE, the Sorbonne, but the students at Reading are having their occupation now.

'Are you in or out, man?

'I don't know.'

'You're a student, so you're in.'

'I'm an artist.'

I tell him I'm an artist and think that means non-political. I'm not a radical, I'm a liberal, I say. I believe in finding some middle reasonable way. But I'm not sure what the students exactly want, apart from wanting to protest.

I go down to the Department and sit at my donkey, plug on with my piece of work. From his corner De Gruyter whistles one of the Brandenburgs. He talks about R.B. Kitaj, with whom he says he's corresponding. I now know the Eliot portrait is an enlarged copy of Wyndham Lewis' portrait of the poet being painted in the style of Kitaj, but that only makes it odder to me. I don't see why he's making a copy. He's fiddling with it anyway, hardly progressing.

Not much is happening with me either. I keep myself to

myself and do a bit of work in the studios when it's quiet. I draw the spider plants in the Victorian greenhouses.

Mmm, colour. The green and white of the spider plants is easy. Green, white and black are manageable. Now of course I'm face to face with it. I've chosen to study art, and colour is everywhere. Actually, I am more worried about how I will fare in art history than in my own art. I can paint any colours I like, but will I be able to study other people's paintings effectively? Will my colour deficiency hold me back? The funny thing is no one knows about it at Reading. It wasn't spotted at my interview. It was more the other way round: my rendering of a Colham landscape, just an oil pastel drawing out of the attic window, received praise for its sensitive handling and colour. It helped secure my place. I'm keeping my Achilles heel to myself for now. Maybe it doesn't matter anyway. That's what I want to think. It isn't my fault, after all – it's a handicap. Lise kindly says it's like Beethoven, which it isn't.

I go up to Bedford to see her.

I seem to be hitching to Bedford most weekends that first term, leaving on Friday morning, returning Monday afternoon. I still hitch by default, never think to take the train or work out a coach route. It's a grim journey that starts on the M4 slip road outside Reading, having taken a bus there or on one occasion trudged there. I get out at Chiswick and struggle round the North Circular to the M1. The North Circular's a bugger for hitchers, all piecemeal, interchanges and broken hard shoulders. I'm dropped in places where drivers shouldn't stop, walk on through the fumes, rain, fog and dark, thumb stuck out; meet other hitchers with their signs and resignation. Then things improve at the start of the M1. There's a permanent queue on this slip road but you do get rides. On occasion great rides in fast cars. How extraordinary it is to come in from hours in the cold, into some businessman's Jag, join him on his journey home for the weekend with Bach on the stereo radio, warm and snug.

It's snug in Lise and Anna's flat too. I settle back into Bedford life for the weekend. Long weekends of walks, food and love. The cinema shows good films. We see Bergman's beautiful *The Touch*, Visconti's *Death in Venice*. Apparently, the portrait Frank took in the garden last year of me in my striped Breton tee shirt is the spitting image of Tadzio in the film. The prospect of returning to my room in student hall and the Fine Art studios is dismal indeed. It becomes worse every time I go up to see Lise. In the end I persuade her to join me in Reading next term. You're meant to stay in hall for the whole of the first year but I will get out. I'll plead misery and get special dispensation. Then we'll rent a flat together in the town.

Getting back to Reading takes most of Monday, a journey which seems a whole lot worse than Friday's, the traffic heavier, the waits for a ride longer.

On one of these returns I got caught up in a motorway pile-up in thick fog on the M1 at Luton. The driver saw it just in time and managed to swerve into the outside lane; we crawled past dozens of shunted vehicles, jacknifed lorries. I only found out how serious it had been in the newspaper next day: seven people killed. Four months later this 'motorway madness' happened again, the same place in the fog: 160 vehicles this time, nine killed.

With the Bedford weekends I'm only at the university for three days a week, but I seem to do all the work required of me. I attend the few lectures and tutorials in History of Art and Sociology, turn up at the studios about twice a week. I'm not asked to produce any specific artwork, am left pretty much on my own. De Gruyter's painting remains on his easel, looking the same as it did on the first morning. He toys with it, whistles and hums snatches of Bach, apparently at work. My own showing for the first term's work is minimal indeed – a few drawings of spider plants and a grey rose on a trellis.

It's already the end of term and there's to be a beano in the studios. A new band called Roxy Music are playing at the Christmas party (it's their third ever gig after Slough Community Centre and the Tate Gallery for Friends). The band originated in part at Newcastle University, which also has a Fine Art course – the one run by Richard Hamilton, on which one of his pupils was a Bryan Ferry. Their sax player Andy Mackay did music at Reading. I hardly remember the gig, I get myself stewed out of my head. There's a much-used 'vomitorium'; I spend a lot of time head against the wall, peeing away pints of beer. Mud (Roger Waters) from our year is carried insensible through the crowd by a statuesque third-year, Polly Eltes, dressed as the Snow Queen. Of the band themselves, I'm afraid I recall nothing. Just a couple of days later, I see, they will play with another new band called Genesis at the Hobbit's Garden Club in Wimbledon, an event hosted by a young John Peel, and be invited to record for his BBC radio show *Sounds of the Seventies*.

I spend Christmas at home at Waterloo Road. Lise joins us – in a photo she's on the floor among my sisters and the wrapping paper. Mum adored Lise, thought her so special, said she could always talk to her. How my mother needed to talk. Lise found *her* special – beautiful, colourful and barmy, she said, and also unfulfilled. She thought my mother was a 'lost' person somehow. I took up with this idea and came to think of her as a woman who had got herself lost in a small Somerset town far from the city where she belonged. It made me blame her less for things.

Now Lise comes with me to Reading to look for a room. I have pleaded with the warden of Child's Hall and got out after just one term. Following ads in the *Evening Post*, we end up in the rough end of town, in the exotically named Zinzan Street. It feels miles from the university, though is actually only a half-hour's walk away. Our Irish landlord shows us a pleasant top-floor room, light, sunny, with a big bed – since Italy we have made do with single beds. The kitchen is shared and grotty; the bathroom is downstairs. The only thing we do to our new room is quieten the 1920s dressing table, which a previous tenant has painted bright orange, with white gloss paint. We spread a pink Indian bedspread over our grand double bed. It's our first flat on our own and we'll live there for the spring and summer terms. My grant is just about enough for two. On Saturday mornings we walk into the town centre to Tesco's in the new Butts Centre, where we buy a French stick and something exotic from the delicatessen. Our little ritual is to tear off the ends of bread while still in the shop.

Lise carries on with her eternal A levels by correspondence. She enquires about enrolling at the Technical College but it's the wrong time of year. She doesn't get a job and is rather in limbo in our room; she's waiting for me when I come home. But often we're both at Zinzan Street during the day. There's a lot of time for reading. We're working through the Russian classics now: Turgenev's *On the Eve*, Tolstoy's *Childhood, Boyhood and Youth*. Lise introduces me to these stories. I love them, so vast and enveloping. With Dostoevsky, I identify more with Prince Myshkin in *The Idiot* than Lise's Raskolnikov in *Crime and Punishment*. We've both read *War and Peace* now. When we were at my father's, Lise asked him what he thought about some of the book's big questions. 'That's the sort of thing one asks less and less as one grows older,' he replied, disappointingly, pipe in mouth, busying himself polishing the floor. What he most loves, it seems, is waxing his wooden floors, scrubbing the stone-flagged kitchen floor till it gleams.

'Your funny family,' Lise says, 'but I so want to go to Colham again. Let's go soon. Show me the wood anemones, the wild garlic.'

Fellow student Pete Hay is living a few minutes walk away in Castle Hill. Pete rarely leaves his room – he doesn't go into the studios at all. He's older and more experienced. He works at home, at night, lives a curious hamsterish existence in the fug of his room, which is in a permanent mess of open books and paintings spread all over the floor; a life partly fuelled by drugs. An alarming character called Catchpole from upstairs keeps him supplied. Catchpole wears a bib and brace and keeps a vibrator in the top pocket, which he brandishes at women. We like Pete, go up to Castle Hill to share a joint, listen to Van Morrison and mournful John Martyn, look at his books on mysticism and mythology. Pete's interests are many, his library of books and catalogues is already extensive: Blake, Palmer, Klee, Paul Nash, Huxley, Leary. Alfred Watkins' ley lines. Frazer's *The Golden Bough*. He shows me the magical formula of the Gnostics, found on Abraxas stones, later used by Daniel Defoe in his account of the Great Plague, and then by Aleister Crowley:

ABRACADABRA
ABRACADABR
ABRACADAB
ABRACADA
ABRACAD
ABRACA
ABRAC
ABRA
ABR
AB
A

Pete loves the young Samuel Palmer and paints Palmeresque landscapes, small, intense, watercolour and ink works from his imagination; he builds them up, scrubs them out, digs deep into the paper. He was thrown out of his architecture course at Cambridge – for taking drugs and not working – but now seems to have found exactly what he wants to do.

'I should say so,' says De Gruyter, still in his corner of the studio with the same painting and his catchphrase. His friend Dave left for Chelsea after only a term but he has a new one in Scottish Al, now ensconced nearby. I stay up at that end too. I'm slow getting to know the rest of my year. Pete never comes in. I'm hardly aware of Dee, another future great friend. There's her friend Margaret, who is getting together with blond Viking Peter already; there's Mud, whose Ben Nicholson-ish scratchings on boards I admire; and Chris already moving into sculpture; and blonde Jane from Norfolk who took my photograph in the greenhouse. Then there are some I never get to know: another Pete, Lorraine, Jonathan ... and my future friend Martin Andrews whom I'm hardly aware of at this time; we'll meet when I come back to live in Reading thirty years later.

De Gruyter gives everyone nicknames. Al is Ludwig on account of his Beethoven explosion of hair; a tall rangy guy with long black locks is Paganini. Ludders and Paggers. De Gruyter can be cruel with his sobriquets: one girl who has rather pointed breasts, or perhaps it's her bra, he names Pneumatic Bliss from an Aldous Huxley novel. But I laugh too at the deadly accuracy. I don't know if he ever gives me a nickname – I never hear one. I had many at school, not all of them kind: Paddington Bear, Squeaker, Auntie Joanie (mercifully shortened to Joan) and the obvious Frog.

There's a sculpture option this second term. I leave De Gruyter and Ludwig in the studio: De Gruyter adding a cat corpse to his painting, Ludwig, hungover, attacking his canvases with variations of Munch's *Scream* and Soutine's bloody abattoirs paintings. I want to make a white plaster relief, something like the interior of Colham farmhouse with its thick curved walls and beams, something like a Ben Nicholson relief I've seen recently. I work my slab of clay and over the next weeks create a clay beam/shelf /mantelpiece with a carefully positioned clay apple, and cast it in plaster. The sculpture tutor Chris Layne lovingly teaches me the stages of making a plaster cast: 'You soap the plaster mould so the water runs off like a duck's back.' Then I work at the plaster with a blade, carving crisp edges to suggest the angles and beams of the low-ceilinged Colham rooms. I'm pleased with the result, the feeling of my white 'Interior Rectangle with Apple', and that's probably my lot for the term so far as Fine Art is concerned.

There are a couple of art history seminars with Peter Fitzgerald and presumably at least one essay that term. Fitz, extraordinarily, chain-smokes a pipe *and* cigarettes, alternately, through his seminars. The room fills up with thick tobacco fug. Up on the campus, sociology and anthropology lectures are more frequent. They also hand out extensive reading lists, Durkheim to Margaret Mead. This ties in with Lise's A level Sociology and we work at these books together. In Zinzan Street we look at extended families in London in *Family and Kinship in East London* by Michael Young and Peter Willmott.

We sit sunning ourselves on the rickety iron fire escape at the back on a warm April day, with Mead's *Coming of Age in Western Samoa*. Lise talks about her two years in Fiji as a child, when she didn't wear shoes except to walk on the coral reef. It's an image that fills me with longing; one day I'll do that too. Meanwhile, we actually look for jobs in *The Lady*, as recommended by her mother. We're after: 'Couple wanted for stately home, cook and maid/duties in house, possibly governess, etc, and handyman for house and grounds; live in cottage; all found.' There are such places to be found on the Berkshire and Newbury Downs. We'd have to say we were married, of course, but 'No children or pets' wouldn't be a problem. We'd have our own cottage and I could carry on being a student while carrying out my handyman duties. We decide too that we'll get a kitten.

Across the road from us, in a basement, lives a Marc Bolan

doppelgänger, a third or fourth year Fine Art student. We notice how late he gets up, watch his curtains from our window. That's fascinating too, this pretty boy in his dirty filthy basement.

A drinking scene forms up at the union bar on the campus. Alcohol is cheapest there, student rate, and you can just about afford to get plastered. I go with De Gruyter, Ludwig and Paggers. Then Lise comes too. Existentialists we are: life is meaningless, existence for mere moments, for this moment only; there never was and never would be any point to it. The graffiti on the toilet walls says it all: TO DO IS TO BE, Kant; TO BE IS TO DO, Sartre; DO BE DO BE DO – Frank Sinatra. Exactly. We drink pints and whisky chasers and the cider beer mix they call 'snakebite'. As in a scene from Sartre's *The Roads to Freedom*, we go round the circle stabbing a knife between our splayed fingers into the bar table. We grip a glass so tightly it must break in our hands. De Gruyter crushes his brandy glass deliberately so it does break. The gash is deep and he's taken to hospital for stitches. Apparently, though I have no clear memory of this, his girl Louise doesn't go with him. It's Lise who accompanies him to the hospital.

One night – it's later, when De Gruyter, Ludwig and Paggers have moved into a flat together, also down the Oxford Road in nearby Waylen Street – we are rolling back down the hill from the union bar in the early hours, when for a dare someone suggests we climb out along the illuminated sign over the new dual carriageway, the Inner Distribution Road. The sign is very much bigger and higher when you are up close to it. I follow the others over the railings, make the little jump across, and I'm standing on a road sign miles above the tarmac. With arms outspread like a tightrope walker – like Philippe Petit on his high wire between the Twin Towers only two years later – I walk to the end. Turn and walk back. Four or five of us do this. I can hardly believe it. Lise watches us. Perhaps it's all about trying to impress a woman. That road sign is still there, and now has a spiked barrier to prevent such pranks, and probably to keep off the graffiti artists too.

Lise's mother comes to visit us in Reading. Lise still can't be seen to be sleeping with me. The ludicrous situation holds sway. We have one room with a double bed, but we don't actually lie together in it. If the thing isn't blatantly in her face, then her mum will be able to turn a blind eye, Lise says. So I move out for the night. I have to empty my half of the wardrobe and take my clothes with me to maintain the illusion. I go round to the house of the reprobate existentialists De Gruyter et al in Waylen Street – what a dive, what a pit. Ludwig is actually drying out his mattress after the girl he plied so heavily with drinks the previous evening wet it during the night. It isn't entirely funny and he knows it as he giggles to hide his distaste and guilt.

There's a group tutorial with Roger Cook. Tutorials of any kind being so rare, you try not to miss them. Even Pete comes in from Castle Hill. Cook bollocks me for not working. He bollocks everyone – no one's doing anything like enough work. My argument, the same since day one and entirely true, is that I can't work from dry in the studios. Any inspiration vanishes as soon as I sit at my donkey. Cook suggests I work outside then, go and find my inspiration. Carry on in the greenhouses, anywhere, so long as I don't sit on my arse saying there's nothing doing. Good advice, as far as it goes.

So, in May, Lise and I get a tent and hitch to the Brecon Beacons. It rains as only Wales can when you are camping. We pitch our tent somewhere just off the road and hunker down. I draw a mountain stream from the mouth of the tent. I watch birds – a ring ouzel – from the tent. We heat up our tins of soup and rice pudding while the rain falls outside. It seems an eternity but is probably only a day.

Back at Zinzan I turn the drawing into a painting of a stylised mountain stream falling from top to bottom of the picture. A slight thing on dark linen canvas with most of the canvas left bare, but I think it my best bit of work so far. Alas, at a second Cook tutorial it doesn't cut much ice. A bit more effort, trial, experiment, boldness, risk and colour, he suggests. But I have a caveat. I'm an Art History student really, like De Gruyter, and I've done enough to satisfy the Fine Art requirements of my first year. I have only to go up to the campus and sit my Sociology and Anthropology part ones to proceed to History of Art with Fine Art next year.

At weekends I go bird watching at the gravel pits on the outskirts of town. Lise comes along a couple of times but it isn't really her scene. Anyway, I soon realise I prefer to go alone – and she probably prefers to have the room to herself for a while. I've joined Reading Ornithological Club and been shown some good local sites. I take my binoculars, the old Greenkats I've had since I was fifteen, and head out to Burghfield and Theale, where there are miles of gravel pits, some partly excavated, landscaped and replanted, others still under excavation. There are masses of ducks and waders, many birds of passage at these semi-urban locations. In the winter, I see goldeneye and smew come down from the Arctic. In early summer, delicate migrating yellow wagtails pause on the gravel of an active pit.

A tutor, Tom Cross, arranges a meeting with the bird artist Robert Gillmor, an ex-student, who is still living with his parents in Northcourt Avenue and working from a shed in the back garden. Gillmor shows me his current work, his sketches and watercolours and linocuts, all of them of birds, a passion and uncompromising dedication to birds, and I can see at once I'm not going in that direction. I couldn't paint like that if I wanted to, and I don't want to. It leaves a bad taste now, but I imagined I wasn't at art school to do 'mere' illustration, no, I would be doing real painting. My thoughts, derived from my father, who was a 'real' artist, did run something like that; they were full of that kind of aloofness. I think the whole ethos of Fine Art at Reading encouraged it too – as if we were all going to end up as self-sufficient artists. I've noticed Gillmor's illustrations ever since, throughout his long career. Above all his linocuts: prolific, consistently good, with a flat and true quality on the page.

On my way into the studios one day, I buy Lise a ring from the pawnbroker's in London Street. We've both gazed at the dozens of 'lost' gold rings in its window. I get her a plain band of whitish gold. 'Oh Johnny, we can't afford it,' she protests and probably we can't. She'll wear it for the rest of our time together, neither of us realising that it's a wedding ring. We have to be told. We're living in our own dreamworld.

Then we go back to Bedford for the summer vacation, or rather to Rushden in Northants, where Lise's sister Anna and her boyfriend Paul have moved. Anna is working in a children's home in Rushden now. She's such a warm bubbly person, Anna, with her laugh and sense of fun. What can I say about her? That she taught me the most basic rule of cooking is to start by frying an onion. When I think of her I see deep red and purplish colours, purple paint generously slopped on the walls of her room or a piece of furniture, a long plum home-dyed cotton dress, and cooking with aubergines which she calls eggplants.

The four of us are going on holiday to Greece, and Lise and I need to get some money together. Lise finds waitressing work as before and I get a job at a furniture workshop. It's seriously hard work. They seem to be producing furniture on an industrial scale. I'm on the end of the circular saw, catching the chair legs as they come flying through. The machine never stops, and you have to keep up with it, catch every piece and stack it correctly. After six weeks of this I've built up impressive biceps and take to wearing a singlet to show them off. I lie in the yard to tan during the lunch break. But I don't get on with the guys working there, and this worries me. I'm not one of them. Only the 'Paddy' is friendly and open enough to come and sit with me. I can see he's a bit of a loser with his shabby clothes and stubble, while he sees that I at least will talk to him. This 'not being one of the lads' will recur. Being a real outsider is different from being an existential one in the Union bar.

Paul has been to Greece before, hitched behind the Iron Curtain all the way to Athens. He regales us with tales of his hitching days, the excitement, the hospitality, as well as how dirt cheap everything is, how you can live off selling your clothes, your jeans, to people desperate for a bit of the West. And then the heaven of Greek islands, taking a night ferry out to the islands, sleeping on deck under the stars. How if you run out of money you just sell some blood, which pays enough to keep you for a few more weeks. This time, though, we'll be driving down through Yugoslavia and round Albania. Paul has bought an old Morris Minor for the job. He spends days doing it up, poking about inside and underneath – I don't have a clue what he's doing. I don't know how an internal combustion engine works. How come men know all this? Do they get it from each other? Not that I can even drive. One lesson with my father among the haystacks at Colham and another with Frank around a disused aerodrome on the Blackdown Hills are the sum of my driving experience, and will remain so until I'm in my thirties. My humble task from Paul is to make an AUS sticker for the Australians, Anna and Lise, to go with our own GB and glue it on the boot.

We don't reach Greece. But we have a good enough time camping in Yugoslavia, dawdling down the Dalmatian Coast. Lise lies in the sun until she gets sunstroke; we cook on campfires and retire to our pair of tents; we see marvellous Trogir and Split, reach Dubrovnik in the south. Then Paul decides that the

Morris isn't up to going any further. So we turn round and take the inland route home, visiting the Bosnian towns of Mostar and Sarajevo, which have such a terrible resonance now. We walk across old Mostar Bridge where the boys dive, then as now, recklessly into a green river pool far below. Twenty years later this amazing ancient bridge, a massive stone span over the gorge that divides the Muslim and Croat towns, will be destroyed by Croatian shelling; in another ten years it will be rebuilt and opened in 2004 as a UNESCO World Heritage Site, and tourists will flock back there. We visit a mosque and look round a Muslim cemetery with its curiously different headstones and grave markers. Lise raves about the intensity of the colours in the 'Turkish' houses; I admire their rusticity. More and more I'm turning to the simple and vernacular in architecture. When we reach Austria, home of the most lavish Baroque and Rococo, I'm as happy visiting a whitewashed Romanesque church high in the mountains as any opulent cathedral.

Strong, invincible Paul gets us and the old Morris Minor safely home. Outside Dover we stop in the early hours at a transport café he knows for a longed-for bacon sandwich. I won't see Paul again (nor Anna). Not so many years later it comes as a great shock to learn that he has died from a brain tumour in his early forties.

4. Macrobiotic

Lise and I arrive back in Reading for the second year with nowhere to live. In the common room of St David's Hall with its sofas and armchairs and a hatch serving tea and cakes, we meet Dee, who is looking for someone to share a flat just along the road. We sign straightaway for 102 London Road, a big improvement on our last place: close to the Fine Art Department, a spacious ground-floor room, grand double bed made up of two singles pushed together. We position the bed in the bay window, unfold our Indian bedspread. But we are signing up for a number of other things by living here in London Road: Buddhism, macrobiotic cooking, being the local drop-in for all and sundry. Dee is like a big bouncing puppy. With her around there's always something going on. We bring our new black kitten Bubby into the mix, too.

My father has come to Reading! By chance he has followed me. From being Head of Painting at Chelsea, he is now Professor of Fine Art at Reading. He rang me up in the spring to tell me that he might become my professor and hoped I didn't mind too much. I said I didn't, though it would probably be the most significant event of my fourth, and as it turned out my last, term at Reading. Of course it'll be all right, having my dad around, I said – just a bit like having my stepfather as art master at school all over again. But I do feel a little queasy every time I walk down the university corridors and either do or don't meet my father. Very recently Dad told me that had I objected he wouldn't have taken the job. Could this be true? Surely it was in the way of his ambition. I was surprised, touched by his concern, but at the time – and probably even now – would never have voiced an objection.

In the abstract/figurative divide now polarising the Art

Department, Dee is firmly on the representational side. As are all my friends, De Gruyter, Pete, Ludwig, Mud. She does portraits – serious, brooding self-portraits – and landscapes. She shows us her recent landscapes propped around her room. She's vulnerable, wants reassurance. All these paintings were done away from the studios without any help from tutors. As soon as she arrived in the new flat she went out to the overgrown cemetery by the Junction and painted its graceful weeping birch tree.

Dee was in many ways a country girl then, up from Dorset and not *au fait* with the smart urbanity of much of the course at Reading. She didn't get on with the tutors hot from London, and they saw her as an out-of-date landscape painter. She was given a hard time at tutorials, and sometimes reduced to tears. Was it really for not being into abstract experimentation? Wasn't it also for being a slightly plump, unworldly girl? They got it wrong. It's the strongest vindication that she should be still painting her portraits and landscapes forty years later, has earned her living by them for many years without recourse to teaching.

I'm on the figurative side too, but I've stopped painting for now. For one thing, art history has fully kicked in after the introductory year and I've realised how much there is to read. With my joint degree I have to both practise fine art and study its history – it's a lot more than I thought. Uncertainly, I abandon the studios and bury myself in nineteenth century European art in the flat. I spread my books on the bed and floor and try to knuckle down. The hectic London Road flat is hopeless for study, especially for someone so suddenly half-sure as me.

Dee hosts the university Buddhist Society under the guidance of Zengo in her room. I attend a few of these meetings, chant my Oms, sit cross-legged and earnestly attempt the half-lotus position. Then Zengo is unmasked. What a laugh to find our impressively robed and shaven-headed monk has been trying to continue the evenings in Dee's bed! Randy old Zengo! Like the Maharishi's stealthy advances on Mia Farrow's sister in Rishikesh, so memorably commemorated in the Beatles song 'Sexy Sadie', Zengo has been unable to prevent himself from taking advantage of spiritual enlightenment.

Tied in with the Buddhism and the general *zeitgeist* is our new macrobiotic diet. Suddenly we are all vegetarian. It's stir-fries, crunchy vegetables with brown rice. We munch through platefuls of almost-raw veg pepped up with soy sauce and tahini paste. And large numbers of people start turning up for dinner. People of all kinds latch on to Dee. She's always bringing home some bod she has met during the day. 'Cosmic Ray', encountered on a train, insinuates himself into the flat. He sleeps for weeks on a bit of floor, and probably lasts so long because he's a good stir-fryer. But in the end dear Cosmic Ray – early incarnation of Neil in *The Young Ones* – gets booted out.

Dee knows another Ray, an artist now living in West Reading. We go over to see his work. Amazing paintings: great dramas of industrial landscape, sky painted as torridly as the land; smoke belching from industrial chimneys and loved for its colour and drama, the way it unifies sky and land – whereas I call it pollution. These large, thick and crusty oil paintings fill his digs in Brunswick Street. Ray Atkins, long out of college, is struggling to survive on his art. He ekes out a living teaching evening classes; he buys paint before food, or so it seems. His rooms are short on the creature comforts. Behind propped-up paintings, hides the bath. A gramophone and classical LPs occupy the only table. There's nowhere to sit down. Doesn't appear to be any heating – just a hungry electric meter. Ray lives on the edge. Of course I'm seeing all this from within Lise's arms, from the comfort of a settled relationship, but it does look bloody uncomfortable. Ray is unconcerned. He's warm and confident. I will get to know him well later on.

De Gruyter, Ludwig and Paggers, who are still at Waylen

Street, just down the road from Ray, begin calling at London Road. They're like a gang now, threatening when they sweep through our 'rice and beans' kitchen in their long black coats. We crunch up our vegetables and troop over the road with them, the existentialists, to the Jack of Both Sides pub. De Gruyter has a car, or access to a car from home – he actually has a driving licence – and he takes us for exhilarating drives. Singing Dylan's 'Oxford Town' we drive up to London on a weekday, race through the West End, park anywhere, check out the exhibitions. It's my first visit to Cork Street's private art galleries. They are free, you can breeze in and out, see them all in an hour. De Gruyter knows his way round. He even buys art sometimes, somehow, one or two original prints – R.B.Kitaj, David Jones, Robert Colquhoun, none of whom I really like. I remember we talk about Kurt Schwitters, whom I do find interesting: 'Merz', making art from rubbish; taking some rubbish and only making 'small changes'.

Lise and I visit Granny Helen in London as promised. On a November afternoon, we find her in her 'small hotel off Sloane Square' where she holds court to her many relatives most years. These may be the rooms where, as family legend later has it, she also entertained Laurence Olivier. While working on *The Rats of Norway*, they'd had an affair. It only lasted until Vivien Leigh came along but they remained good friends. It seems their friendship continued, much of it by letter, right through to the 60s. My father, in another of his *aperçus*, suddenly remembered that his mother once had a flat behind Oxford Street, where he stayed when he was twelve (this would have been 1938), and the actor would bring his son, aged seven or eight, for Helen to look after for the day. 'There was a knock at the door and there was Olivier with his son. Often.'

We have warming tea and cake with Helen in her chintzy suite. She gets on as well as ever with Lise, and when I settle down to read an archaeology article in the *Telegraph*, she remarks, oddly yet pleasingly, that I'm 'turning into a character'.

The London Road flat becomes ever more chaotic. Our unhousetrained kitten doesn't help. The loo now has a notice pinned on the door: BUBBY'S BOG. No one washes up, the sink fills up and up, clogs with grease and is abandoned. There's too much mess now to even contemplate a start. It's an essay in decrepitude, very *Withnail and I*, with Bubby thrown in. *Withnail* is some years off, but it will strike a common chord amongst us students of the 70s. Are student kitchens still like this? Is living in a state of absolute squalor perversely enjoyed by everyone who goes to college? It gets so bad we have to hang out in St David's Hall common room with the newspaper and a plate of eggs and chips through the hatch – so much for the macrobiotic diet.

Walking along London Road to the Department one day, deep in leathery autumn plane leaves, kicking them up, ploughing through the piles, Lise and I pass the pretty boy who gets up so late in his Zinzan Street basement. 'You make such a beautiful couple,' he says, charming us, and while being flattered, it also somehow sets off alarm bells with me. We aren't as close as we were. A bit routine, a bit stuck, unsure of where we're going. Yet Lise is ever more popular among my friends. I remember something De Gruyter said about my building Lise up in his mind as this wonderful creature before she even came to Reading, and then when she arrived how she really lived up to being that special woman, the centre of so much attention. Perhaps she has as much to say to these guys as she does to me now, and especially to De Gruyter.

Terry Frost has come to give a talk on colour. De Gruyter groans, resolute in his anti-modernist views, but we all go along. It's a Fine Art lecture and introduced by the new professor, my father. After the mild discomfort of having him speak in front of us all,

Dad melts away and Frost takes over, inspiringly. He illustrates his talk with his own slides of boats and lorries and women in summer dresses; the world as he sees it, all juxtaposed shapes and curves and strong colour. His enthusiasm is ferocious and infectious. But he's an abstract painter, and so it seems, inevitably against us, the figuratives. Though Dee and De Gruyter are worlds apart in their own figurative work, they find a common battleground here. Terry Frost is just shapes on a canvas, and very big shapes at that. Where is the substance and *meaning* in it? After I leave Frost will become a regular visiting tutor at Reading. One day he suggests De Gruyter turn his canvas upside down to see its formal values. You can imagine what De Gruyter thinks of that. Now, I would say that Frost was right to talk of the painting in those terms, but he might have been missing De Gruyter's interest in literary values and symbolic meanings.

There are modern art history lectures too, by Brian Petrie, whom De Gruyter approves of, and Caroline Tisdall, whom he has reservations about. Especially when she champions Joseph Beuys, who has exhibited a wedge of lard on a chair to represent the human condition. I knew nothing about Beuys' life then, his great survival story – how his bomber crashed over the Ukraine in the war and he was found by nomadic Tatar tribesmen who covered him in animal fat, wrapped him in felt and saved his life – and how all his art has become informed by that. Not knowing this, I tend to agree with De Gruyter that lard on a chair isn't art. It can't be art just because you say it is … how deep the water is straightaway: isn't that exactly what the brilliant Marcel Duchamp, every art student's hero, said over fifty years ago?

Actually, our Fine Art year, with its mix of figurative and abstract painting and sculpture, is mostly quite traditional, at least it's 'plastic' (and concrete). More radical and avant-garde are the years above. The new 'isms' are in Film and Live Art, in Installations and Happenings. Fourth year Anne Bean is a major offender. For instance: as part of her degree show she will present a piece entitled 'What is an Artist?' in a stinking wooden fish box. It isn't accepted. A performance by her art school band Moody and the Menstruators – a private performance given to four examiners on a sofa – won't be accepted either. For Anne everything she creates can indeed be called a Happening. And there's suddenly masses of this stuff around. Bruce Lacey is in the news this summer: dressed up as a Red Indian in a tepee in Hyde Park; performing an 'At home' installation with his family in a tent. Installations. Happenings. They're about anything, complains De Gruyter, advance for advance's sake, no rules, no traditions; where does it all come from? We tend to go along with De Gruyter. We don't get Gilbert and George's 'singing sculpture' *Underneath the arches* performed on a table; Stuart Brisley with his *And for Today – Nothing* performance: lying in a bath of black water two hours a day for two weeks while the wash basin beside him filled with offal, decayed, flies laid their eggs and maggots hatched. It doesn't seem to relate with anything we're doing. So influential on me is De Gruyter's rubbishing of this experimental art that it will be years before I can look at it afresh.

I go back to Fitz's smoke-filled room. Amid the bone-dry Neo-classicists, I find the early Romantic Géricault's *Raft of the Medusa* a powerful contrast. Géricault, I notice, also made a prescient series of paintings of the mentally ill: *Portrait of an Insane Woman*, *Portrait of a Kleptomaniac*. Like the English Romantic poets he died young, aged just 32. Through the clouds of smoke in the seminar room there's beautiful Polly, the girl who dressed as the Snow Queen at the Christmas party, the girl who, I hear, is in Anne Bean's outrageous band. Polly is majoring in History of Art too. She doesn't say much in the seminars, but then nor do I.

The fascinatingly named Moody and the Menstruators – who become known as the Moodies – are a loose-formed group, founded, Anne says, for anyone in the Department who wanted to be in a band. They are sparkly, camp and decadent. The line-up varies but always seems to include a lot of lovely women. Talented keyboard player and singer Rod Melvin is in it, and sometimes the Marc Bolan lookalike from Zinzan Street. The rest are women. Becky who has sunbathed topless on the lawn, Polly who now haunts my art history seminars.

Inspired by Pete and his love of English Romantic painters, I make a trip to the Ashmolean in Oxford to see the Samuel Palmers in their special collection. They are brought to me at a table, in a folder, in their cardboard mounts, unframed. I hold in my own hands these original ink and watercolour marvels. So small in the flesh, so fine and densely worked.

We aren't seeing much of Pete now. He's still in Castle Hill and doesn't get up to London Road – he doesn't get up, period – but late that autumn he leads a trip to the famous Wittenham Clumps. He shows me a Paul Nash painting of the clumps – the beautiful, mystical *Landscape of the Moon's Last Phase* with an enormous lumpy yellow moon sinking behind the twin wooded clumps. These hills have other names: Sinodun Hills, derived from the Celtic; Seno-Dunum, 'old fort'; the Berkshire Bubs (this was just before the county boundary with Oxfordshire was redrawn); Mother Dunch's Buttocks – you can get all this information online in minutes now, but it's just what Pete would have stolidly researched on his own through the night.

I'm not sure whether Lise comes on this trip. And it isn't De Gruyter's cup of tea. Dee, Marg and Mud are there, I remember. We get up and catch the bus at lunchtime to the town of Dorchester, no mean feat for a bunch of students on a frosty December day. From there we set off for the distant clumps. It's a long way, the last part through ploughed fields of sticky clay, and we don't reach the top until dusk. But this is all for the better as we see them by moonlight. The night is clear and cold, frost settling on the leaves and earth. It's exhilarating and mysterious, mystical if you like. We walk back through the muddy fields with clodded boots and shoes. The last bus to Reading has already gone, so we repair to the pub. Later in the evening we hitch home in the back of a stinking butcher's van.

Then it snaps with Lise. I suddenly know it's over. Something has been constricting, holding me down. I can't see where I am any more. I seem to be losing myself. I tell her I want to leave, don't have any idea where to, just leave, and she collapses. Then I collapse. Our world of two and a half years falls apart just before Christmas. We started so young. We've had so little experience in relationships, have so little to go by, but just seem to have run dry. We aren't going anywhere any more. The wide bed with its pink bedspread sees hours and hours of talking in circles, nights of tears. Does my father's presence have something to do with it, too? Perhaps. I don't know. I go to my new tutor Tom Cross in tears and tell him I'm leaving the university. He strongly disagrees with this and tells me to go home, have a rest and see what the New Year brings. In pain and bewilderment, in sorrow and emptiness, I see Lise off on the train to London with Bubby the cat. We meet Pete on the platform in a porter's uniform – his new temporary job. It's an odd little encounter. He is sheepish, we are at the world's end. He doesn't know we are splitting up and we don't enlighten him.

Lise has gone. The doctor puts me on Valium. The small yellow tablets, which I recognise from Mum's pill saucer at home, knock me into a state of numbness. My father drives me down to Colham for the Christmas holiday in a back-seat blur. Madeleine, the farmer's daughter I fancied in my early teens, and who is now at Reading University, is getting a lift home too. I can't speak to her from my clouded head and just sit through the long journey in silence.

Lise goes to her father's too, in London, and then to his remote cottage in Wales. Just after Christmas, she writes me a long letter, descriptive of the landscape, 'the tawny brown hill' opposite her window, where you can walk twenty-five miles and hardly see another house, and how it's the last stronghold of red kites in Britain. She says our Bubby is with her and not pregnant as we feared. She agrees that we should split up and re-start our lives. We've stopped being good for each other.

5. Out in the world

I lie in bed in the attic at Colham, foetal, catatonic. I see her face all the time. Her face close up, her eyes. I'm shattered. We hurt each other – all the things we said. I hurt her more – I broke us up. We were hurt and we got ill. I have butterflies thinking of her. I mustn't think of her. My father has brought me hot Marmite. No whisky and lemon hot toddy, his catch-all remedy for colds and anything else, as I'm on these drugs and he doesn't know how they mix. He sighs and sits on the end of the bed. I'm back in my tiny childhood room. I'm lying there telling him there's no point in anything – you know the kind of thing.

'Die in harness,' says Dad, getting up and pacing about. 'That's what was once said to me, and I've always rather stuck to it. Not such a bad philosophy for life. We just have to carry on, really.'

This doesn't make much of an impression at the time. It hardly dents my armadillo shell. I need to know whether to take another breath or not. A kick up the arse from him might have done better. But his words have lasted. Yes, to die in harness is just about the best way of looking at it. I've become an advocate of the go-on-till-you-drop way of life, use up every last bit of time you're given. Perhaps another reason I remember this scene with my father pacing about the attic, is that it was one of the rare times he had actually mothered me since I was very small and my mother wasn't around to do it. It was the only time in my adult life I fully collapsed on him.

It's New Year. Awakening. It doesn't take so long. You are still grieving but can look ahead too. There is a future while you grieve. In another letter Lise said she'd be going back to Reading, to London Road. I might see her.

It's January, 1973. I decide to leave the university but return to Reading and get a job. I do find Lise in the flat and there's even some attempt at reconciliation. We take a while to move out of London Road; we sleep together again once more, one last sad night. You need the physical contact as much as anything. A relationship ends and suddenly all the sex has gone, no wonder you feel empty. But there isn't to be any going back.

I look for a houseshare with Mud and his girlfriend Karen. We find a two-up two-down terrace in the aptly named Little Street, sign the rental agreement with the landlord Mr Zieba – £8 a week, it seems so much – and move in. I have the small upstairs bedroom at the back of the house. It's actually my first room of my own. House-proud, I buy a can of Dove Grey emulsion from Woolworths and paint the walls. My bed is about ten yards from the railway tracks, the main Great Western line, and the night-magnified sounds of every train entering and leaving Reading station.

But Little Street is a much-needed oasis. I get on with Mud who works on his textured, scraped boards, arrangements of landscape and seascape forms; a St Ives-influenced painter. He comes from Saltash and will eventually go back that way, with Karen, and become an art teacher in a Cornish school. He introduces me to the then firmly Labour *Daily Mirror*. We also take the *News of the World* on Sundays to play with the headlines, composing ever more absurd collages of sex romps on the vicarage lawn. We do the *Mirror* and *NOTW* crosswords together.

I take a job as a trainee landscape gardener for Waterer's. Gardening in midwinter is tough. The early morning start in the dark comes as a shock to my flabby system, especially when I know the others in the house won't be getting up for hours. Loss of the easy student life rankles and burns.

Mud keeps me up to date with the Department. There's been a tragedy: the Chinese guy, jilted by his girlfriend, has hanged himself in the studios. It was my father who found him when he went into work early in the morning. Dad didn't tell me about this for years and years. How terrible it must have been for him.

Then another shock. Lise is going out with De Gruyter. Didn't I see this coming? There were surely clues at London Road, the drinking sessions, the madcap drives in his car, but I hardly registered them. And when it does happen, I must say, I react badly. I become deeply jealous. I'm not aware how much this shows until one evening, at a John Lill piano recital in the Town Hall, I see them together in the foyer and turn away in a whirl of confusion. Lise comes up to me, furious, tells me I'm behaving appallingly; I should grow up. Indeed, I lack the social graces. I try to avoid them after that, as I know I must. I have to find someone too.

I go to discos in the student halls – those discos disdained when I first arrived at the university – and learn to dance by imitation. Santana's 'Samba Pa Ti' is creaming away at Wantage Hall one night and I'm dancing with a girl maybe called Verity. I go back to sit on the floor of someone's room, a loud girl called Shane, who has a bevy of girls around her, and we drink Southern Comfort, listen to Neil Young's *Harvest* and Van Morrison's *Tupelo Honey*. Another night at another hall down in Kendrick Road I get lucky. I dance, well, bop, seem to do all right out there on the dance floor, and approach a blonde girl from the Art Department whom I've hardly spoken to before and find she's ready to dance with me, and go to bed afterwards. She takes me to her room and strips off without inhibition. Which enables me to strip with the light on too. That piece of graffiti humour on the toilet walls of the time comes to mind: I thought cunnilingus was an airline before I discovered a certain brand of vodka. This is good, all I want, but in the morning I'm required to leave. My first true one-night stand: just a lot of sex and off you go.

I start going to the Union disco on Friday nights with Mud

and Karen, bop with them, bop by myself, thumbs stuck in the belt loops of my jeans, shaking my long hair. Ludwig is there with a smuggled-in bottle of whisky, yelling the Nilsson song: *Can't live if living is without you* … We bob and jive to 'Whisky in the Jar', and, innocently, to Gary Glitter's 'Do You Wanna Touch Me'. I love the wildness of the Stones, the exhibitionism of David Bowie. I find myself in front of this slim girl with a boyish pageboy haircut. I think she's dancing with me. I'm edging in and, yes, we are definitely dancing together. Some signal passes between us and now we're clasping hands, pulling each other back and forth, away, round, and rubbing back to back like cats. I hardly know what I'm doing but she responds to every move. It's there, sealed. 'What's your name?' 'Mandy.' 'John.' We bop on to 'Brown Sugar': *dance just like a black girl should*, and 'The Jean Genie': *he's outrageous, lives on his back* … The chemistry, that's what they call it, is working again. We stay together for the rest of the evening, then go back to her room.

Mandy and I get on fine and our Friday nights become regular. Her place is just off the campus, and I meet her in the disco and go back with her. I'm not her only partner, I realise, but I don't mind that too much. She's promiscuous and so am I. It's just sex. The two bodies that meld together so well on the dance floor are the same in bed. I love her gamin body and almond eyes. Then in the morning I avert my eyes from the Beatrix Potter prints on her walls. Did she put those up? I don't think I even enquire. I don't think she's serious about me either, she doesn't want it to be complicated.

But I must get up in the mornings and this will be my undoing. At 7 a.m. Reg is waiting in the Waterer's van somewhere in West Reading. While everyone lies in their warm bed sleeping it off, I set off to work at a run with a grabbed sandwich and flask.

Reg and I cover the 'rhododendron belt' from Bucks to West Berks to Surrey. There's a surprising amount of gardening to be done in the winter. Reg is very different from me. A tiny man but wiry, much stronger than me; only forty but he has no teeth left and mumbles unintelligibly. I do the *Mirror* crossword he can't do while we sit in the van for our mumbly lunch breaks. We spend one week laying a great lawn in Sunningdale – it was next door to Diana Dors' house – and I scrounge the leftover turf. Reg says it's fine, 'waste not', and drives me back to Little Street that evening. We stack the turves on the pavement; I lay a lawn over the whole of our tiny patch of garden by the railway tracks.

But I continue to be late in the mornings and am eventually sacked for keeping the van waiting. It's like the trouble I got into at school for getting up late, a perennial problem which will last until I'm into my forties and begin to wake up early naturally. I don't mind losing this job, though. It's a relief and a spur. I've been making my plans. I have a bit of money saved now and am going out into the world to investigate. I've volunteered for an archaeological dig and as a warden on two bird reserves.

6. Ospreys and redstarts

In April I set out in my new Doc Marten boots, hitch up to the dig in Shropshire and spend two weeks in a field on a freezing hilltop. There's a Roman villa under the claggy earth, every bit of which is being removed in buckets for sifting on a trestle table. It's painstaking work and there are no great finds, no coins or jewellery, just a few shards of pottery and tile – this is archaeology, not treasure hunting; we are aiming to plot the floorplan of a two-thousand-year-old house. There are a dozen volunteers at a time and we lodge at a hostel in Telford. After our day in the field, exposed, windburnt, suffering from a surfeit of fresh air, I at least happily spend my small daily pocket allowance in the pub. I make friends with 'Gilbert the Filbert', a student at the Institute of Archaeology in London, a lively and eccentric chap with a passion for his subject, for everything Mortimer Wheeler has done for archaeology. He gives me a contact for a dig in Tuscany, which I will follow up in the summer.

On my last night we go to *A Clockwork Orange* in the local cinema, where it hasn't been banned – we catch that brief period of general release before Stanley Kubrick has the film withdrawn following an incident of copycat violence. It's a deeply shocking film with its juxtaposing of ultra-violence, including sexual violence, and Beethoven – and I've hardly been able to listen to the Ninth Symphony since without some echo of those truncheon-wielding, milk-drinking Droogs. *Orange* will remain withdrawn, unseen, until Kubrick's death twenty-seven years later, and a measure of its power is that I could remember it all when it was finally shown on television.

Next day, heading home to Somerset through the Welsh borders, I experience some of the loneliest hitching of my life. Lifts peter out, it's miserably cold and wet. At dusk I find a ruined house by the road, roll out my sleeping bag on the floor and crawl into it, supperless. I wake up next morning, alone and breakfastless, to my twentieth birthday and get back on the road.

A few weeks later, fed on the milk and bananas of home, and having called in at Reading to see Mandy, I'm hitching off to Loch Garten on Speyside, as an RSPB volunteer on the first osprey nest protection scheme. It's a long journey, a hitch of a couple of days of which I have little memory, but I do the last part by train in order to be met at Kingussie by the warden and get a lift to remote Loch Garten. Base camp is deep in the Abernethy Forest, a last remaining part of the ancient Caledonian forest of Scotland, in large army-style tents with a caravan field kitchen. Living among a group of keen young naturalists you get to see a lot. There's so much more around than I ever realised. One morning a flock of exotic waxwings pass through the camp on their last hop north to Scandinavia. There are crossbills in the Scots pines, crested tits and red squirrels on the feeders, and of course there are ospreys every day. We cycle on pine-needle paths through the deep quiet of the forest to the osprey hide; work on shifts through the day, talk to visitors, note the activities on the osprey nest through a powerful pair of binoculars bolted into the hide. I've brought a sketch pad and materials with me – soft pencils, chalks, watercolours – but hardly have time to use them. I go off one morning and make a drawing of some silver birch trees, but generally there's too much else going on. I keep a bird diary: *Male capercaillie, 7.45 a.m. on the road, cycled right up to him. Huge black bird with shaggy beard. Eight-mile walk in evening over moors from Glen More Lodge looking for peregrine.* I also record some of my impressions. In a page torn from the back of the RSPB osprey logbook and kept in a future journal, I find the following account of a day. It has an idealised best-of-all-possible-worlds tone – a very special day and night I wanted to preserve in amber – and was written during my night watch in the osprey hide while my fellow watcher slept.

16 May 1973. The alarm went at 7. Stumbled from the tent into a beautiful sunny morning – like those early spring mornings in Italy two years ago. I was on early watch. The ospreys were quiet, the female sitting well down in the nest with only her head visible, the male perched on his usual dead branch in the next tree. The 40x binoculars pick out every feather, the fierce eyes on constant alert for danger; these rare birds sit there unaware of their importance, this great protection scheme set up for their benefit. Visitors began to arrive at 10, school groups, families, couples. Everyone took a turn to stare through the big binoculars, trying to connect with the distant specks in the two trees, fumbling with glasses and their own binoculars; some went away disappointed, others happy; the 'knowledgeable' were disdainful of the amateurs around them. We're supposed to talk to everyone but there are too many people at once, and they don't stay long.

Cycled back to camp for lunch. Warm, the forest quiet and still, full of light and shadow, floor a spongy mass of rich green and brown tones.

In the afternoon a trip up the Cairngorms on the back of Alan's motorbike. We took the easy way to the summit with the chair lift. An icy wind on top. Snow. Dazzling views of snowy peaks all around, a pure green loch below, blue haze over Spey Valley and Glen More. The snow was melting fast in the sun and water ran off in all directions, exposing ground bare except for mosses and lichens, with granite boulders sparkling. We didn't see a single bird in two hours.

Back at camp for a few hours rest. Then we set off for the night watch. It doesn't get completely dark until 11. The wind dropped, the sky was clear. It was a full moon night and the ospreys were asleep in their trees. I took the first watch: a red grouse scolded, a cuckoo called, deer barked, tawny owls called. Dark for only three hours, dawn breaking behind the osprey eyrie at 2.30. The male was visible on his perch all the time, the female we could hear through the microphone shifting about on her nest.

My stint with the ospreys of Loch Garten lasted only two weeks. It seemed so much longer. From there I went to Coombes Valley in Staffordshire, another RSPB reserve, for a month. The mere six weeks I spent in these two places seem to contain a disproportionate chunk of my life.

I have a lift from Speyside to Newcastle, leaving at 4.30 a.m., so there will be time, in true birder fashion, to squeeze in a visit to Flamborough Head on the way. The North Yorkshire cliffs are a fantastic spectacle at the height of the nesting season. Then my companion drops me at my road and I hitch on alone to Leek. 20 *May. Sunday. Hitching hell after rainy night in leaking tent. No money or food. Found skylark's nest in grass on a roundabout (4 eggs).* I arrive at last at the warden's house on the edge of the moors above Coombes Valley. Morris takes me down to the volunteers' cottage I will be sharing with three others. It lies deep in the wooded valley of the reserve, rudimentary, without electricity, and it's a little paradise. The timing of late May is 'Perfick', as one of my new companions says, as they do in *The Darling Buds of May*. We wake to a fanfare dawn chorus in the morning and make our porridge on the calor gas stove. The birdsong is a symphony all around us. Morris comes down, warm and jovial, and sets us to work on the reserve for the day. Thus the days pass, clearing paths, scything bracken, coppicing, fixing a plaque on an oak stump, monitoring the nest boxes, showing the few visitors to the reserve around. The valley teems with birds, residents and summer migrants, a host of warblers, cuckoos, nightingales, flycatchers, which can all be identified and traced in the thick woods by their calls. Wood warblers sing their shimmering song near the house, and are easy to see as warblers go. The equally lovely willow warbler cascades are everywhere. A pair of piping kingfishers visit the pond to fish and we watch them from the hide; the female has a red lower mandible, the male a black one;

such minutiae are there to be learnt. Marvellously, we go out at dusk to watch ghostly nightjars flit among the treetops and the strange woodcock's 'roding' display, circling a glade at speed, croaking. For a change of scene, Morris takes us over the Peak moors to see a black grouse 'lek' and then a herd of escaped, naturalised Tasmanian wallabies – they are still living there and now on the British mammal list.

I'm adding species to my own 'life list' of birds all the time. Mapping the nest boxes, I find a redstart inside one with seven turquoise eggs, then a pied flycatcher with chicks, both new species for me. I encounter a sparrowhawk dashing low through the trees – I've never positively identified one before. I catch a young grass snake in my hands and am squirted with foul-smelling liquid. Someone brings in a young tawny owl for Morris to look after; he's always being brought injured and orphaned creatures to be saved, he sighs. We go out owling in the night, following the calls of tawny and barn owls and the 'hoo hoo' of rare long-eared owls.

Settling down at the cottage, I get out my sketchbook. It's a full-time job working on the reserve but I want to do some drawing too. In the evenings, even the early mornings with a cup of tea and the dawn chorus, I work on several quite elaborate studies in chalks and watercolour of the view from my window. On a day off, my bird diary says, I spend seven hours painting. Thus I fill a small travelling sketchbook. Looking at these pictures now I see how derivative they are of my father's work at Colham. Or you could say connected. For this place fills me with the happiness of that Wiltshire valley.

Someone comes to film the badgers. This is fascinating to watch, and I see just how long it takes to get any results at all: biscuits dipped in honey at the entrance to the sett; locating a place to film from, a tree in this case; then perching in the tree for hours night after night. It's a job that combines iron tenacity with infinite patience. We volunteers are allowed to creep to the site at twilight, downwind, and observe from a distance – while being bitten to pieces by the midges. And the badgers do come out, they snuffle and trundle around eating the biscuits, before we retreat to our midge-free house. I've often remembered that filmmaker and believe he became well-known at the BBC Natural History Unit working on the Attenborough *Life* epics. Maybe he was Hugh Miles. Loch Garten and Coombes Valley marked one of those turning points in life. I could have followed my nose and pursued my interest in natural history as a career. But I didn't. I moved back towards art instead. My landscape drawings were what I brought away with me from the cottage in Coombes Valley. And I'd decided to do some more archaeology, in Italy this time.

Suddenly I'm back in Reading, where I still have a toehold at Mud and Karen's in Little Street. I take the bus out to the sewage works at Manor Farm – a good birding spot – sharp with my new knowledge, and, gratifyingly, am able to identify a green sandpiper, ruffs and bearded tits among the reeds around the sludge pits. This sultry summer's day on Reading's reeking waste is among my best birding days to date.

In the time I was away Mandy discovered she was pregnant and had an abortion. Not by me. She says it wasn't me and I don't know whether to believe her. The abortion was recent but she allows me to stay with her. She's very laid-back about such a monumental event, and even allows some gentle lovemaking. I'm happy to be with her again, imagine we might stick together, Mandy and I – the Peter Rabbits on the wall notwithstanding. But when I get back from Italy at the end of the summer, it's obviously over. She has gone home to Yorkshire, and we haven't made any plans. We write to each other once. She wishes me well 'above and below stairs'. I'm so grateful for her openness and sheer joy of sex.

At the Union, to which I still feel I belong, Anne Bean's Moodies are competing in the Battle of the Bands. I get to see this mythical band at last. And I'm entranced: the bravura, outrageousness, sheer sexiness of the singing girls. Such a beguiling mix of posing, dressing up, and soulful pop. They do 'Itsy Bitsy Teenie Weenie Yellow Polka Dot Bikini' as a cabaret act, and then Rod sings a deeply soulful 'Help Me Through The Night'. They are in competition that night with Clayton and The Argonauts, the band of future prolific rock music writer Ian Clayton, whose existence I'm unaware of at the time; he was even living a few doors along at 92 London Road the previous winter.

The Moodies win. Afterwards, I find myself sitting beside Polly on the lobby floor. I've seen her there, back against the wall, long legs stretched out, and gone over, or maybe she beckoned me over. Anyway, here we are, side by side, brushing shoulders, and she's asking what happened with my art history. Why did I disappear, quit the course? She takes sips of my beer as we talk. I tell her about my plans, for Italy and archaeology in the summer, and her close attention, her sipping from my glass, thrills me. I go skipping home across the campus that night. Polly has invited me to visit their place any time.

The Bean house is a tall Georgian townhouse in Southampton Street. I see only the ground floor, but it's as extraordinary inside as I imagined. On a hot cloudy afternoon, I climb the steps to the front door, knock sweatily. Ridiculous to be here, to have taken up this idle invitation. Someone ushers me in, and I'm shown, rather formally, round a few den-like rooms: black rooms, festooned with sheets and cobwebby things, curtains drawn, mattresses everywhere; a night house. Polly isn't in. I don't see her, and in fact won't see her again. I stay for a cup of tea and learn that the house is coming to an end. Degree shows are over and everyone's moving up to London, to a squat in the East End. My tea, like some kind of interview for life's lottery, comes to an end. I stumble out into the bright daylight with relief, yet that black house will continue to interest me for years.

Hitching up to London to see my new archaeologist friend Gilbert, standing in line on the M4 slipway, an old ambulance stops. Anne Bean again, the happening artist – and here's another Happening. She waves to everyone on the road to climb in the back, she empties the road of hitchhikers, which is so cool of her. The ambulance trundles up to London and goes straight through the middle, dropping us off as we request. I go south to a flat in Balham and find Gilbert the Filbert sitting in the middle of a chintzy living-room floor in a Moroccan jelabi, smoking a curved pipe of something, holding court to a group of friends who evidently adore him. I'm also smoking a pipe now, off and on, combined with my roll-ups. I enjoy the grip of the briar between my teeth. Next day Gilbert takes me on a tour of the Institute of Archaeology in Gordon Square. In the basement, he carelessly picks a small Egyptian arrowhead from a pile and gives it to me. 'It's all right, it's a broken one.' One won't be missed, he assures me, but still this is a shameful bit of pilfering. Gilbert suggests that I come to the Institute and become an archaeologist, too.

I might do that, but not now, for I've heard they want me at the summer dig in Italy. In early July, a month after leaving Coombes Valley, I'm hitching off again to the earthquake-hit town of Tuscania.

7. Among archaeologists

I arrive in Tuscania after a forty-eight-hour hitch and very few hours' sleep. The June heat of Italy has sapped me. I get ill and take to my bed in the dormitory. I'm worried about my finances. My new travel diary details how extraordinarily little money I have, how little I started with – only £12 left after I'd bought my ferry ticket.

On the night boat from Dover to Ostend I joined up with a happy-go-lucky sort from Leeds whose luggage was what would fit into his boiler suit pockets. He was going to Germany to work. We found ourselves a ride with an Asian guy who said he'd take us all the way to Cologne, at crazy speed, overtaking on the inside lane, the hard shoulder, which left me feeling sick and slightly hysterical. But our lunatic driver got stuck at Aachen on the German border with an untaxed car and we left him there up shit-creek, thumbed on our separate ways. There were many others on the road, crowds of summer hitchers traversing Europe. Small camps with smoky fires and guitars had sprung up in corners away from the road. 'Wuppertal, Wuppertal!' a young German was yelling, high on something, as he ran up the slip road to the autobahn. The police came by and picked him up. He had long hair, was probably on drugs, would be in trouble. All friends out there on the road, we defended him, united in our hatred of Authority. The police, the pigs, cruised round like sharks on the lookout for any excuse to nab us too. '*Scheisen, scheisen*,' we yelled.

I picked up rides, moved south. At the Karlsrühe interchange I walked into town to buy some food. I went into a cheap-looking bar for a beer. It was dark and blissfully cool inside after the heat of the road. Oddly dark, with blue and red lights. I sat down and sipped my beer. A woman approached me, put her hand on my leg and asked if I wanted anything. 'Nein, nein, just a beer, bitte, danke!' I got back to the autobahn, rolled out my sleeping bag among some bushes and slept for a while. This was the same route I had taken with Lise two years before, the same way south. I was on my own now, but that was okay. I could handle this. I hitched on after dark, crossed through Austria into northern Italy overnight. *On the way to Orvieto at last. Very happy, no fears or worries*, I scribbled in post-lift euphoria after a long day standing by the road somewhere in northern industrial Italy and at last getting that big lorry ride every hitcher dreams of.

I didn't reach Tuscania that night, but slept on the beach of nearby Lake Bolsena. It was magical: stretched out on warm black volcanic sand, a yellow moon in the sky and the croaking of frogs. Then waking to the most perfect early morning, a mist hanging over the still viscous surface of the lake, everything pink as the sun came through the mist, the silhouettes of fishing boats like gondolas, a standing oarsman slowly drifting past. *All alone on the black sand, alone and free* ... I write.

Fellow archaeologist Ralph keeps me company in the dormitory. Ralph is marvellously lazy. He's not ill but 'acclimatizing', not quite ready to go out into the burning sun to dig. He tells me about Tuscania, hit by a massive earthquake two years ago and still in ruins. The basilica of San Pietro high on its rock survived but not much else did, and the town is now the subject of archaeological investigation. There's a medieval town, a Roman town underneath it, and then an Etruscan one under that.

Digging in Tuscania is pretty much as it was in Shropshire, a matter of scraping off a layer of earth, collecting it in buckets, sifting it on tables, bagging and labelling absolutely everything that might be of interest. Only this time it's in broiling sun. An American guy who looks like Jack Nicholson refuses a sun hat and gets his face badly burnt; I watch his temple redden and turn livid as he patiently prises at the baked earth. We start early and work until it's too hot; have lunch, a siesta, and take the rest of the day off. In my free time I wander off with my binoculars and see some new birds: red-backed shrike, Sardinian warbler, golden oriole. I make a drawing of the basilica, stark earthquake survivor perched on its rock, in red and black chalks.

The evening meals are boisterous, with much wine, but I find myself at a loss at the dinner table. These people are different. My solo hitch all the way from England seems very odd to them. It's something none of them would do and marks me out in some way. I become more aware of this as the days go by – what's everyone so damn jolly about here? They're so *easy* socially. I get plenty of thumps on the back to jolly me up but that only distances me more. The outsider, I struggle to join in with these insouciant archaeologists. It's money, isn't it? Money and a bit of class. But this is silly of me. They are perfectly good people, I'm sure, even if they do have more money than me. No, this mood emanates from me. I ward it off by going birdwatching and sketching alone.

A letter from Frank finds its way out to the dig.

Dear John
You had a letter from Clare this week, otherwise we have neglected you. Mum is off letters though she is fairly well. Catherine is in bed with measles and feels really ill. Her face is swollen and she has a high temperature. She was due an illness, I think, as she has been overdoing things for some weeks. Babysitting, a steady boyfriend, ballet, guitar, etc, and the prospect of being confirmed!

Clare has got a place at the Slade Hostel, which is what she wanted. Sarah is busy collecting nettles for a big cage of tortoiseshell butterflies she is looking after for school. Granny is weaker and keeps falling down.

I'm glad you have been doing some painting. That's more than I have. I could easily give up painting for good and probably would if I didn't teach it. My creative ability is small. The recorder and chess still fill all my spare time, except for sporadic gardening. Scotland must have been enjoyable, getting up at dawn and so on. Thanks for the cards.

The car has been very expensive lately – shock absorbers and brakes. They take all your money and are a damned nuisance.

My latest idea is to buy a second-hand tape recorder (regardless of the last paragraph) so that I can play duets with myself. Also Catherine wants to hear herself sing. And I suppose we could tape things from the wireless.

Mum loves getting cards from you and of course sends her love. She says she can't write at present.

All good wishes from us all.

Frank, so reliable, reassuring, keeping you up with the news. Frank, looking after everyone's needs at home – Clare, Catherine, Sarah, Mum. Where would we all be without him? Modest man, he has this low regard for his own art. He regularly loses faith in his abilities and threatens to give up on 'these little weekend paintings' but he never quite does. Solitary man, he plays duets with himself. His latest craze with the recorder is taking over from chess, and he will excel at it, as he did with chess at the school club. He always asks me to write to Mum, 'however short'.

I write back that all is fine. That's what I post. An unfinished card says rather differently. It starts off saying I'm feeling down and blue, finds there isn't enough space to explain this, and is abandoned. Well, you don't want to write home about not having a good time.

But there are good times among the archaeologists, too. A visit to Etruscan tombs, crawling inside the unfenced tombs by torchlight. An expedition to a ruined medieval village that turns into an adventure, when, trooping through scrubland in torrid heat, we encounter a great horned bull on the path; we retreat, detour, tread single file through snaky grass, over crumbling walls into the village, which has almost totally returned to forest. It's fine doing things like this. I get on with Ralph and the sunburnt American and a woman called Caroline who has generously invited me to use her apartment in Rome if I'm down that way. What I can't manage is the after-dinner table, sitting around telling endless jokes and stories. This must be me, surely. Has something got into my head that wasn't there before? I writhe and berate myself, constantly pull myself down when I'm among these people. I just want to escape – am I getting depressed? Some alarm bell in my head tells me this is the reason for my isolation; people don't like to get too near the depressed.

My month at Tuscania will soon be up, but I'm not going home yet. I'm not ready. What's there to go back for anyway? I hear of another dig in Umbria. Someone in Assisi is desperate for a volunteer. I put in for the job and get it.

I go via Rome. My daily pocket money, saved to a lump sum at the end, provides enough to take the train and spend a couple of days in Rome. I can stay in Caroline's empty apartment. I love it there, so 'simple and Japanese', though Caroline herself is thoroughly expatriate British – she works at the British Council, just part-time, to supplement a private income. I sleep in the big bed alone, go out into the blaring horns of Rome, trek round the sights. The Sistine Chapel, which my father first showed me at the age of eight, in all honesty I still find dark and distant; more overwhelming than the work itself are the shuffling crowds, the heat and stuffiness of incense. So much has been said and written about the famous Sistine ceiling, but it was almost invisible in the years before it was cleaned. Yet I'm deeply moved by Michelangelo's *Pieta* inside the entrance of St Peter's. It strikes a note with my own insides, connects with my mother somewhere. The Madonna has a wound of her own – she was attacked with a hammer a year ago by one Lazlo Toth crying 'I am Jesus Christ'. What I'm looking at now is the remarkably quick restoration, already back in place and behind new bulletproof glass. Apparently, witnesses to the attack made off with the broken pieces as relics and treasures, and though most were returned in then end, her nose never was.

I write letters home. I write to Lise for our good times in Italy, I want to tell her I'm having a good time. And to Granny Helen to let her know that I'm planning to visit again on my way home. And to Dee in Reading. The teas and Buddhist artefacts in the apartment remind me of Dee's kitchen at London Road; I tried to get into her bed after breaking with Lise and failed.

'Feel terrible. Hope I'm not getting ill,' ends my brief Roman diary.

'You were,' it scrawls in reply.

Now I'm off to work in a monastery, taking the train to Assisi, transferring at Foligno to a little chugger with wooden benches. A bald rangy man with gold NHS glasses and a most earnest, charming manner meets me at the station. I feel better already. I'm so glad to move on from my solitary Roman holiday.

Hugo is doing a PhD on a cache of medieval majolica discovered in the walls in the Basilica di San Francesco and he needs two draughtsmen for the summer. Richard has just arrived from the V&A. I told Hugo on the phone in Tuscania that I could do the job but I had little idea. I plucked up and went to see draughtsman John for advice – John, most socially oiled, most Wodehousian of the chaps who so alienated me – and he encouraged me, said that archaeological drawing was a doddle, far better than sweating it out on the dig itself. One-to-one, I found he wasn't such a scary person. Again, my fear of his easy social graces was due to my lack of them.

The monastery at Assisi is magnificent and vast, built on top of the famous church filled with Giotto's frescoes, which are now in the vaults. (This of course was before the great earthquake of 1997, when the church and half the monastery collapsed and the frescoes were buried.) It's a very active place, home to scores of monks, whose cells are arranged in tiers around the central colonnaded courtyards. Sheer walls rise from the cliffs on one side, and from the windows of the room where we work there's a huge view that stretches from the neat monastic kitchen gardens far below to the modern town of Lower Assisi and out across the plain – a view from deep within the monastery which few outsiders see. The draughtsmen's tables are set up at these windows. Our job is to make drawings of the more important pot segments in the recent find. My first piece of eleventh-century painted majolica is ready waiting. I think of John's drawings in Tuscania, the detail, the dead accuracy of scale, the plan-, side- and cross-section views, all carefully inked in. I glance across at Richard's drawing already under way … get the hang of it in the end but am a tortoise. Hugo is disappointed to discover my evident lack of experience, but he's a patient man; I'll just have to knuckle down and learn. I do okay in the end, but doubt I was worth my weight in pocket money.

Each day we break at noon for lunch, and what a lunch. At first we eat with the monks – rowdy, jovial, *long* affairs, and I'm reminded both of school dinner times and of the joke where the monks have heard the stock jokes so often they no longer need to tell them, just give the number, and everyone laughs. Then our lunch is brought to us in our own dining room, and it's substantial. Pasta is just the starter; there's a separate meat course, salad, fruit, wine … but no siesta. After an hour of eating, we must stagger back to the drawing board to give Hugo his money's worth.

Our lodgings are in an apartment in the town belonging to one of the 'outreach' padres. It's a pleasant walk home in the evening through quiet cobbled streets, now empty of tourists. And we get on well enough, Hugo, Richard and I, well enough for a month. When Hugo hears me stumbling over answering the dreaded question 'What do you do?' – Nothing. I'm not at college, not in a job, not working for my career – he comes to my aid. 'Just say you work in a bank. That keeps them quiet.'

There isn't much free time – there's always another pot to draw – but zealous as ever of my own time, I get away when I can to explore. Assisi is indeed a lovely place: the old hilltop town of white stone, the vineyards and olive groves around it. The sky is cloudless day after day. I walk and stop to sketch in the shade of an olive tree, hear nightingales loud in a thicket during the day, and the fluting calls of golden orioles; I see the weird and wonderful crested hoopoe. Yes, what's there to be heavy-hearted about? Nothing, nothing at all. I walk on, get to know these winding medieval Assisi streets, come across the convent of Santa Chiara. The order of Saint Clare is, fascinatingly, silent. The woman in shadow on the other side of the grille never speaks. Can this be true? She must talk with the other nuns, surely. She must talk to herself. I tiptoe away in awe. I love the frescoes of St Francis feeding the birds, and find the whole story of his life and relations with Clare beguiling. It seems to me they were obviously in love, but diverted their love through you know who.

One evening Hugo, Richard and I climb to the summit of Monte Subasio and sleep out. We set off at sunset. As the sun goes down a full moon rises exactly opposite – it always does. Brother sun and sister moon, Saint Francis and Sister Clare. We walk up to the Carcere, St Francis' hermitage, where he retreated late in his life. It lies in a fantastic position among thick oak woods at the head of a valley; five hundred years ago small passages were cut out of the rock, four-foot high doors opening onto small hewn-out rooms with a little window looking over the plain. It's dark when we follow the only path up through the woods to the top of the mountain – high above the black plain speckled with lights and immense sky. We walk along the thistly, herb-scented top in the bright moonlight, eat our dry bread and cheese. Lie down to sleep on a slithery slope at 4,000 feet, a cold wind getting up. Between snatches of sleep I watch the moon cross the sky and count nine shooting stars. At dawn we see the magnificent view for the first time.

'Seen my latest?' Helen is showing me the pictures on her walls again, her new acquisitions. I've turned up on her doorstep a second time, hitchhiking home from Italy, impecunious again – you probably shouldn't do these things twice. 'It's by Stephen Buckley. D'you know him?' I look at the neat little canvas and bamboo construction. 'There's something about his work that's just right,' she says. 'Proportion, clarity, simplicity. I think he's very good. He went to Reading too, for his post-graduate (and in twenty years will come back as Fine Art Professor). How's your painting getting on? How's art school?'

I'm sleeping up at the *Four*, alone this time and very conscious of it; I have a big unposted letter about Assisi to Lise in my bag. Helen shows me her own recent work. She's working on a series of large paintings of tennis players: flat, 'hard-edge', semi-abstracts of stylised leaping figures, rackets, ball, net. Helen amazes me again with her accomplishment. She's painting for her own exhibition now.

Then, at dinner on the terrace, she comes out with this shocking one-liner about Dad's painting: 'Hopeless painter, your father. Should've stuck to his History.' Tully echoes the sentiment. I can hardly believe this – all Helen's prowess flies straight out the window. However great her life story, her accomplishments, her wealth, it won't atone for what she has just said about her son. And actually she's wrong. He's by far the better painter if we're going to take the gloves off.

She asks about Lise and sighs. They got on so well when we turned up on her doorstep two years ago. They got on when we called at her hotel in Sloane Square. She thinks I've really lost someone special in Lise, and I feel to blame for losing her. Then she lays into my mother. Blames her, somehow, for 'succumbing' to mental illness, for not standing up and doing battle with her inner demons. Granny Helen is not in a good mood. This second visit to Biot is turning into a disaster. I realise that I'm involved implicitly in this attack on my mother. Helen has noticed my low spirits, which I'm doing my best to conceal, and she isn't at all sympathetic. I'm succumbing too. Actually, her attitude is similar to my father's, I realise, when I was drifting drugged around Colham last winter and he told me, now famously, that it was better to die in harness rather than sink into listlessness.

But my grandmother hasn't totally given up on me. While the aristocratic Tully snoozes in his armchair after lunch, a fine copy of *Ulysses* open at an early page on his knee – 'He doesn't *read* it, he always falls asleep!' – she points me towards Proust. The world, she says, is divided between those who get on with Proust and those who don't, and she wonders where I will stand. I know nothing of *madeleines* then, but I will take them with me from Biot.

I have pieced together some of Helen and Tully's fascinating story, their wartime escape. Some came from Helen, some from my mother years ago. Recent things are from my father. And when I at last met my Aunt Pagan, around the millenium, she filled in some more.

Granny Helen was the actress Helen Spencer on the London stage when she met Tully. She was doing well, had worked with

Laurence Olivier (in more ways than one). She was also Mrs Froy, married to WAF with two sons. She and WAF lived on the Pevensey Levels in Sussex, in the village of Herstmonceux (good French name), 'right by the old castle and Greenwich Observatory'; the boys, Dad and Nigel, went to boarding school in Eastbourne. Dad remembers the Herstmonceux house as a very romantic place with huge views over the marshes to the sea. He learnt to ride a bike on the long bumpy drive. There were tennis courts. On a visit from school, he saw his future stepfather Tully playing tennis there with his mother, and 'knew'. WAF was at work in London at the time.

Helen left WAF for Tully and they lived at 'Tullens', as they called it, just a few miles away. Tullens was a grand place given by Tully's father, Major Grigg, a wealthy man and owner of 'The Car Mart' on Piccadilly (now the Hard Rock Café). 'He gave all his children houses,' says Pagan. My father, now visiting his mother and new stepfather, remembers they always kept chickens, their 'cawks', they called them.

At the outbreak of war, Granny Helen, the actress, volunteered to entertain the troops in France. Tully volunteered too, as an ambulance driver – 'Because it was easy,' Helen said – and extraordinarily they went in Tully's father's Bentley. It was the time of the Phoney War, there was no fighting yet. Then, as the Germans advanced, and the Allies retreated to Dunkirk, they fled south in the Bentley. 'It was tomato red with wooden running boards along the sides,' says Pagan, five years old at the time and for some reason with them. Her brother Lyn, aged two, had been left in England; Helen was now pregnant with their third child, Hippo. They reached the Riviera and stayed with a friend, 'the lesbian', at Mandelieu-la-Napoule outside Cannes. But the war followed them. Pagan remembers them listening to the wireless, always talking about De Gaulle; she was learning French. There was bombing on the beach where she was swimming. 'I saw a biplane, an Italian plane, approaching over the sea.' Next day they left in the red car with their lesbian friend ('Helen had a thing about lesbians') and drove west to Perpignan. The friend suggested they go on to neutral Portugal, and maybe she did that on her own; there's confusion over what happened to the Bentley and its driver. Helen's family took the train north to Bordeaux, a very slow train; Pagan got off to pick flowers when it stopped. They managed to find a boat full of Polish wounded ('they had walked from Poland') and got back to England. Then spent the rest of the war in Wales and the West Country, moving from house to house with Tully's new job as a munitions inspector. When my father visited them at Machynlleth, he was instructed to stay the night at the station hotel. Next morning Helen and Tully arrived, theatrically, on horseback and they all rode up to the house high on a mountain. Later, while training for the RAF in Plymouth, Dad visited their cottage near Lynmouth, impressing his young half-sister Pagan with his uniform.

After the war Helen and Tully bought 'Uckfield', their chicken farm, with proceeds from the sale of The Car Mart after Major Grigg had died. Apparently Tully was cut out of his father's will because he refused to testify against his mother in court during his father's divorce. Which perhaps puts Tully's ban, forbidding Dad and his brother contact with Helen and their children, more in perspective. The chicken farm did well and eventually they sold up and returned to the south of France in 1958.

I don't get the train fare home this time. I was almost banking on it. But you probably can't do these things twice. Tully takes me to the start of the autoroute, complaining loudly about hitchhikers, all filthy and wet and lighting up their foul tobacco the moment they get in the car. Which must mean me too. He drops me off at the start of the Autoroute du Soleil and I will never see him or Granny Helen again.

I join the line of hitchers, hold out my PARIS sign. A French girl gets out of a car, all tousled ringlets of black hair, and starts to thumb beside me. Sylvie is going to Paris too and says she'll get me a ride. She's friendly, lovely; her shoulders are deep-tanned, breasts loose under her singlet. A car soon stops – for her. It's a lift all the way, a five-hundred-mile ride, but with only room for one, ha ha. Sylvie apologises and scribbles her phone number in Paris.

It takes me very much longer to get there. I reach Lyon after midnight and have a long trudge through the city. I stand on the outskirts for the rest of the night. Then at first light I get a great ride too, all the way. A young couple in a 2CV stop and I climb onto their mountain of baggage in the back. They explain that they aren't using the autoroute because of the toll fees, so the journey will take longer. I lie on the clothes and bedding and the little Citroën trundles slowly across France. I feel acutely the closeness of the couple driving to the city to set up a new home.

In Paris I ring Sylvie from a Metro station and she invites me to her apartment. She'd arrived the day before, amazingly quickly. Her lift turned out to be with some *putain*, she gives a little French shrug, but he was no problem in the end. She shows me where I can sleep and I unroll my sleeping bag on the floor. The moment comes as to whether we are going to sleep together, the moment passes. Was it up to me at all? I have a new timidity– it has been a while, you get out of practice – but besides this I recall some sense of honour: You're just crashing at her place, it isn't an invitation to her bed; she would have asked you if she'd wanted, wouldn't she? All the same I dream about her breasts, her mane of hair on the pillow. In the morning the question remains unasked but perhaps she appreciates my 'discretion' as we whisk up our bowls of hot chocolate. Then she's going to work and I'm leaving, direction home already. I visit the Marmottan in the Bois de Boulogne, as Helen suggested. I'm astonished by Monet's huge waterlily paintings, see some famous Van Goghs in the flesh, but am now more interested in Cézanne's formal treatment of a landscape in terms of the cone, the cylinder, and the sphere. I passed his famous motif, a hazy white Mont St. Victoire at Aix, while pursuing Sylvie up the autoroute. I don't go chasing back to her apartment.

8. Colham intermezzo

My sisters are still on their summer holiday at Colham, and I go straight there to join them. Dad says he loves the Monets in Paris, and anything by Cézanne, but Van Gogh less. I tell him about Biot but not what his mother said about his painting – I never do tell him that. I walk with teenaged Clare and Catherine, separately, in the valley. Clare is now definitely going to the Slade in the autumn. She became quite a star at Taunton at the end, winning a prize for her large abstract painting (it will soon be hanging in Exeter University). I don't actually 'get' this work of my sister's, its flat shapes and beige colours. I don't know, I prefer the little hand-embroidered spider, so detailed and beautifully made, she gave me as a memento. Catherine, nearly sixteen, loves horses and has long golden curls tumbling down her back. She's just getting herself out of her marooning at the local comprehensive, a victim of the all-or-nothing injustice of the 11-plus system, and will soon be on her way to Taunton Tech to do her A levels. According to Frank, both my sisters were in fact borderline with their 11-plus and had to be assessed: Clare passed her interview assessment and went 'up' to grammar school, Catherine stayed down and went to the comp.

It's interesting that Clare is going to the Slade, where both our father and mother went in the late forties. Already, Clare has had no end of it from Mum. Mum was taught by 'Bill' Coldstream and had the time of her life at the Slade. She met our father there. Dad doesn't say much about it as usual. Only recently in his old age has he opened up a few chinks on his private life, some more small illuminations. For instance, having coffee with him one Saturday morning, he said, 'Giacometti came to the Slade once and quite liked a picture of mine.'

'Really, Dad! That's amazing.'

'He singled out three students' work, including mine.'

But it was still down to a Google search to find that the great Alberto Giacometti visited the Slade in 1955, when he was in London for his first big retrospective at the Tate. The critic David Sylvester brought him there, where he met Coldstream and was given a tour of the school. Giacometti remarked on the 'landscape' of easels, donkeys, etc, in the Men's Life Room, which reminded him with pleasure of his own student days at Bourdelle's *atelier* at La Grande Chaumière. He was enthusiastic about the Antique Room with its groupings of Greek casts, skeleton, plants and plaster busts, and the drawings of a student, Martin Froy.

But enough of all that, as my father would say. How about a bit of caustic soda-ing? It's on today's schedule and I'm going to help. Dad has an old cupboard he wants to strip back to the wood. Just as he loves polishing, scrubbing and cleaning things in the house, so he can work this transformation of a piece of furniture, make something really special out of very little, if its core is good.

The cupboard is outside on the gravel under polythene. Just 'junk', cheap pine painted with thick old cream gloss. But he knows it isn't junk. Not when you get back to the original wood. He has this new way of removing the paint with caustic soda, more finely than with a blowtorch or paint stripper. And as ever with Dad, it starts with the preparation, the right equipment, an emphasis on safety: this is outdoor work with a hose run from the kitchen tap, buckets, broom, soft brushes, rubber gloves, gumboots. We mix a caustic solution – just a fleck burns the skin – brush it on, leave it to soak, then hose it off, rubbing at the loosened paint. Several times. We keep hosing and rinsing, slowly, gently – don't scrub, scratch or scrape! Patience! The work will take several days. Warm cloudy August days. The giant hogweed that has self-seeded in the old mill ditch by the house will loom ever higher. Hogweed is a severe irritant, can be dangerous if the spores are ingested, but it's a fine, sculptural thing too; artistic qualities win over caution and the plant is left to grow. We continue to brush on the caustic soda, dissolving away the paint, working down through the layers to the original wood. Little by little the lovely pattern of the wood grain appears. It is soft and vulnerable, easily torn in this wet state. We leave it outside a day or more to dry.

The finished piece is then left as it is, without wax or varnish. It pales as it dries, the wood in perfect condition with a lovely patina. All the finished pieces in the house – a kitchen sideboard, dresser top, table – have been left *au naturel* like this. They are treated with the reverence of art objects. The whole process of stripping furniture with caustic soda becomes part of my artistic training, my sisters' too. When the cupboard is fully dry, we wheel it inside on rollers, my father now dramatizing the event as though we were rolling a great sarsen stone to Stonehenge. Over the threshold, along the boards, into position. The new piece is added but how will it work with what's already there? Dad steps back to scrutinise the intruder through pipe smoke. If the room looks cluttered now, then out something will have to go. He is quite ruthless about this. There's no quarter for clutter in his house.

The bleached, silky, stripped pine cupboard is installed in the sitting room and survives. A plaster sculpture by his friend James Towers is placed on top. It sits there nicely. And it becomes a laugh, a bit of comedy – for the sculpture with its suggestive and ambiguous form comes to be known as The Bra or Towers' Arse. It's still there on top of the cupboard, in another house, another sitting room, with my father in his old age. The pine, though darker now, still looks good.

'John, cut us some chard, will you?'

'Right you are, Pa.'

Swiss chard or 'perpetual spinach', a new vegetable in Britain, grows a metre high with great fleshy white stalks and deep 'iron-rich' leaves. The spuds I also dig for supper, spuds galore fresh and pearly from the black earth, are the best I've ever tasted. A marrow sprouts gigantic from the compost heap. There are carrots, turnips, beetroot, leeks, cabbages, runner beans, French beans, rhubarb, goosegogs. The Colham vegetable plot, a large square in the garden, a *parterre* (Pa-terre), has become a *tour de force*, with marvellous crops growing in the rich valley loam. And food continues to be at the centre of the Colham holidays. If cooking is the heart of the home, then home is here at my dad's.

Dad has a thing about steak. It has to be very good or not at all. Restaurants can never cook it well enough for him – the first steak I ever ate, aged about eight, was with my father on a day out from boarding school, when at a table with crisp white cloth and serviettes I learnt to choose between well-done, medium and rare, learnt about the bloodiness of steak. To cook steak at home he'll drive miles to buy the best fillet from a few butchers dotted about Wiltshire and Gloucestershire; once, the story goes, he crossed the Severn Bridge and went all the way to Abergavenny to get it – surely there must have been some other reason for the journey too. We might have this revered steak once in a holiday, no more. Its excellence is complemented with plenty of wine. Dad never goes for posh wines, says his vino is your ordinary plonk, but it's as well-chosen as the steak. *Vieux Ceps* is a favourite everyday red.

The silence, that Colham mealtime hush, is less evident now. There's a baby in the house. Little Francesca is in her high chair and making a healthy racket. But the silence is still there, still *background*. And isn't it, if you are feeling a bit unsure of yourself, really quite intimidating? Thinking back to those silent heavy meals of our childhood, weren't we in fact always scared of our father as we ate his delicious meals? The way he would push back from the table after the meal and slowly light his pipe, appraising us. View us through the billowing smoke with a raised eyebrow – the raised family right eyebrow – and slowly, desperately slowly, suggest someone fetched the sweet jar to the table. Then he would recite the story of the monkey and the sweet jar again: where the monkey stuffed his greedy paw into the jar, filled it with sweets and wouldn't remove his clenched fist, not even when the hunters came and cut his hand off.

Some nights there's a cabaret after supper. Then there's noise. Chairs are pushed back and we take to the 'stage', the raised area of floor at the end of the dining room. Taking to the floor to do a charade after supper at Dad's has always been a holiday treat – earnestly acted out, with full dressing up and props, as is only fitting for descendants of actress Helen. And we do our music pieces. I strum 'Blowing in the Wind' and 'The Times They Are a-Changin'' and sing with my sisters. I struggle through 'Spanish Romance' on my ropey old guitar, my only classical party piece for years. Catherine H, who is more musical than any of us, plays the piano. Her piano arrived at Colham some time after she did and was installed on the dais. Although she plays well, it's hard to get her to perform solo, she is so modest and deferential. She prefers to be an accompanist to, say, Catherine's singing. My sister has revealed a good folk voice and gives us 'Scarborough Fair'. Yes, we Froys after a good supper and bellyful of wine are a lot of show-offs on that stage, especially our dad. One night he recites T.S. Eliot's *The Love Song of Alfred J. Prufrock*, his very favourite poem. I've come across it before with De Gruyter in Reading, but this is the first time I 'see' the poem. Dad reads it very straight, in an almost normal voice, managing to be both playful and serious at the same time. It's an experience which resonates with me for years.

I get a new classical guitar. I've been managing with my old folk one from school since I had to relinquish my share of Lise's simple sweet-toned guitar. When we were in Bristol, Lise and I lusted together after the 'real' classical guitars in the window of the Spanish Guitar Centre in Whiteladies Road. Now I hitch there from Colham and buy one. £37, I believe, plus £5 for the hard case. I don't know where I found this considerable sum of money.

The day turns into something of an epic when my lifts run dry on the way back. I've just hitched all the way home from Italy but can't manage the twenty miles from Bristol. Stranded with my guitar at dusk on the hilltop by the village of Marshfield on the A4, I ring my father for help. He doesn't respond at all well to this: 'If you're going to hitchhike, then finish the job. Don't think you can just call and get yourself bailed out.' As severe as his mother in France. I'm expecting too much from him. But I have my new cedarwood guitar in its red felt-lined case safely home. I settled on a flamenco guitar with its lighter, harder sound. It is beautiful. I love its tone, which works well with folk music too, love its pale brown colour and cedar smell, and it will accompany me back to art school.

Catherine H will buy a classical guitar from there too and we'll work on duets during the holidays. Handel's jolly *Harmonious Blacksmith* becomes our Colham party piece. We work at Gaspar Sanz and Fernando Sor, and we just about manage the start of the Prelude from Bach's *Cello Suite No.*1 transcribed for guitar. It's a joy to play music with another, more than twice as good.

But at Colham I'm just passing time. I have no more plans. I'm twenty and still don't know what I'm doing.

9. Dark autumn

In the autumn I go to London. That's what you do when you don't know what to do: go up to London. I get a room, get a job, and stay until Christmas.

My first place lasts less than twenty-four hours. I may have spent the first night in London on Clare's floor, smuggled into her Cartwright Gardens room, where she has only just arrived to start at the Slade – or quite possibly I arrived from Somerset on a morning train and had my own room by nightfall. Anyway I buy an *Evening Standard* or *News* and follow an ad down to Peckham. It's a basement and pleasant enough, looks out on railings and the ankles of passers by. The landlord, who lives on the premises, warns me about bringing back 'young ladies'. If I do, I'll be out on my ear. That evening I invite Clare down to see my new lodgings. We go for a drink and something to eat, and Clare comes back to the room to stay the night rather than cross town alone. Next morning there's a knock on the door. I remember protesting my total innocence, that it's my *sister* who has stayed, but it falls on deaf ears and I'm out.

I call Mark Fry, who is now living just up the road in Camberwell. As ever his situation is rather different from mine: he has the top-floor flat in a house that belongs to his family. There's no spare room but he can put me up for the night. I haven't seen him since Florence; he's still with his same girlfriend Anne. We smoke some dope, talk and laugh, old friends – this sounds too casual. I do 'smoke', but only when the stuff is around; I don't keep my own supplies or go looking for it. I smoke other people's dope when offered. Mark is decorating now for money, doing up this very house among other things. He is interested in the more specialised kinds of decorative work such as marbling, *trompe l'oeil* marble fireplaces. It's easy, a piece of cake, he says.

You don't need training, can get it all from books, pick it up as you go along. I could work with him. But the prospect doesn't appeal to me. No, that isn't what I want to do. I remember my interview at the art school just down the road, getting in. I still have that to hold on to. I wonder about trying Camberwell again, perhaps I could rent a room here. We smoke some more. Mark picks up his guitar and plays songs from his new record. He made that record in Rome after all – *Dreaming with Alice* – though it hasn't yet been released in England. He has a beautiful, plaintive voice.

I get out my *Standard* again and by next evening, following the trail of ads in the classifieds, hopping back to North London, I have another room, a grotty place in Turnpike Lane. My first job, also picked from the paper, is packing shirts in C&A, Oxford Street, which lasts three weeks. Then I move to Harrods' wine cellars, a temp until Christmas.

There's an extraordinary world beneath the Harrods store, a dark mirror of what's above. 'You're right under the Brompton Road now, mate.' I walk to work through a maze of subterranean 'streets' where hundreds of people are working by yellow sodium light, by flickering fluorescent light. Forklift trucks and buggies whine their way around the people and goods. There's an invisible staff entrance direct to this underworld and there's a back way to the staff canteen at the top of the building, where I go for lunch – a good discount, my one square meal of the day. The staff world is enormous but it never touches that of the customer. We subterraneans can be there all week and never see the shop. Harrods is still a big deal. It's still the days when you can get Anything there. 'Christian' the lion cub was bought famously for 250 guineas in 1969 (he was eventually returned to the wild in Kenya and survived); California Governor Ronald Reagan was given a baby elephant, Gertie, for Christmas in 1967 by the son of the exiled King of Albania. And so on. News of exotic visitors filters down to us below: sheikhs, actresses, pop stars. One lunch break when I've escaped upstairs into Knightsbridge, I see the tall figure of Pete Townshend, looking somewhat uneasy by one of the entrances.

I discover now that just a few minutes away from my underground world, on 17 November 1973, William Burroughs was having lunch at David Bowie's house in Oakley Street. Perhaps when I was walking down Oakley Street late that afternoon in the dusk to the Albert Bridge to look at the river. Mum lived in Oakley Street at the time of her divorce in 1958, when I was five. She had taken a room by herself and was 'having a go at living alone again'. My sisters and I were being looked after by nannies at the time.

The work is fulfilling customers' orders for Christmas, and for me entails tracking down the wine, single bottle or case, and bringing it to the counter to be packed. Sometimes I pack the parcels. We take our 'tea breaks' among the wine mountains, the dizzying stacks of wooden crates and cardboard boxes. Most take their lunch there as well; they don't leave the cellars until it's time to go home. There's a little nest area, a table and seats of wine crates, where we all drink wine. Sensibly, it's permitted to have a bottle on the go. We smoke too – I doubt that is. I probably go some way towards acquiring a wine habit during my three months in these cellars, and I'm sure most of the permanent staff are too well looked after by the booze to ever want to leave: captive workers for life. We sit down for our morning break, play a round of whist, light up, and pour ourselves a glass of good Burgundy.

I acquire the nickname 'Eric' from one of the other Christmas temps, this dapper young chap called Ken. 'Morning, Eric,' he chirps. 'How's the world treating you?' 'Oh terrible, Ken,' I croak. Ken comes in every morning with the *Telegraph* tucked under his arm and puts his energies into skiving off work. He manages somehow to avoid doing a stroke of work all day. There are many hideaways among the cliffs and canyons of boxes. I find him in some nook and we push in the cork of some vintage with a thumb – there are corkscrews around but they are not an item to carry in your pocket, to be found when you are searched at the cellar exit at the end of the day. Drinking outside break times is also a step across the thin blue line, but it goes on. Fine wines, crudely opened, are being covertly swigged all day. We always drink red, perhaps because it's winter. Wines we couldn't afford, which we could never buy on our modest wages.

I glug a delicious *Fleurie*, warm and fruity in the underground heat. My friend with looks up from his crossword and *Mouton Cadet* and asks: 'Oh, what are we going to *do* with it, Eric? Tell me the grand plans for your life?'

Well, don't ask me! I'm up a blind alley. I spend the hours of daylight in a cellar and go home to my room in the dark. I suffer the rush-hour tube, endure the eternal four minutes between King's Cross and Caledonian Road stations on the Piccadilly Line, the unexplained stops, sometimes with extinguished lights. I walk through the leaf-slush and litter of Turnpike Lane to my lodgings above a shop. In through the back, past the bins and dog bones on the floor, brave the Alsatian and simmering meat bones on the hob. The French wife of the shop owner is always boiling up bones for some stew or stock. Smells of the cooking meat and fat and marrow bones permeate the building. Yelling too from their rooms, frayed tempers and, I think, the occasional blow. Upstairs in my room I light the old 'candlewick' gas fire and sit on the rug in front of it. This becomes my home comfort: to sit close to the softly roaring flames, toast a slice of bread on a fork. I eat my takeaway kebabs and steak pies by the fire. It's all a far cry from brown rice, stir-fries and tahini. Meat is what's available on the street, and it's cheap.

There's another lodger in the next room, a genial and eternally optimistic Brummie, whose ambition is to sing in a band like Robert Plant of Led Zeppelin. He scours the classifieds of the music papers, follows up any ad for a lead singer, comes in to tell me how he's getting on. I'm not much interested in 'Plant' and his stories from the *MM* or *NME*, in all those big rock bands of my youth – Pink Floyd, Led Zeppelin, The Who, the Prog Rockers – but I listen anyway. He's not much interested in Leonard Cohen, Bob Dylan, Neil Young, Joni Mitchell. He doesn't listen to classical music at all.

October turns to November and rolls on to December, the hours of daylight grow ever shorter. At weekends I sometimes go to exhibitions, and I walk down Green Lanes – that maelstrom of buses and jammed traffic – into the relative haven of Finsbury Park. I take a North London Line train round to Kew Gardens, pay my penny at the turnstiles (now £16) and discover the great glasshouses. The small twin Stoke Newington Reservoirs are within walking distance of my room and I'm pleased to find smew, diving ducks which have come down from the Arctic for our warm winter and are uncommon anywhere in Britain let alone inner London. I meet Clare in her lodgings – such comforts! – visit the studios to look at her work, still don't really understand her abstract paintings.

And I go back to Camberwell to see Mark in his freshly-painted black flat – black all over, the ceiling too. Like the Rolling Stones' 'Paint It Black' of years ago, like Anne Bean's house in Reading, like Biba, the new huge 'black' department store in Kensington I've just poked my nose into. We smoke again and this time it doesn't work for me. I'm not laughing any more. The flat downstairs is free that night and I sleep there, have a bad night of it. I suppose I've had hints of bad trips before, seen how it might suddenly all go wrong, turn into some hugely exaggerated nightmare, but this is a real lesson to me. I have crossed the dividing line, narrower than I thought, between fun and paranoia. I lie in bed in terror, utterly alone, convinced I won't last the night. Doubtless this was just a reflection of my state of mind at the time, but I will avoid cannabis and grass for several years now, and then only take it in secure situations.

In November, Mark invites me to a private view in a gallery in the King's Road, where his band are playing. How different from my world now, the world that has closed in around me with my crummy job. My friend has got his own band, has made a record in Italy. I go straight from work and find Mark is busy, of course, with his gig. I don't see much of him. Moving around the fringes of the show, I bump into Anne Bean, with Becky the sunbather. Anne has one black shoe and one white shoe, which I remark on inanely. She tells me the Moodies are still more or less together, they've been to Germany. They're living in a squat in Poplar in the East End, and I should come over. I say I will. They don't stay long, they are bored, I can see. On their way out of the smart Chelsea gallery, Becky nicks a poinsettia; she takes the potted plant from under the gallery's nose and puts it under her coat. 'For the house', she winks as they disappear into the night. I don't follow up Anne's invitation. I think about it for a while and reason my way out of it. Not really me, is it? All too wild for me. I don't have the time anyway, working my five-day, knackering week. I justify myself just as I did over the intimidating black house in Reading. No, I don't want to go into all that again. But part of me knew, obscurely, contrarily, that I was turning down some chance to grow, discover something new about myself, by not going out to Poplar.

I dance to Mark's band for the rest of the evening, then go home to Turnpike Lane, and it's the last time I see my old best friend for thirty-seven years. Our worlds have moved just that bit too far apart. Then they'll roll together again. When I've written these words in the autumn of 2010 and good chance has reunited us.

There's a long letter from my mother in November. I know instantly from the large scrawl on the envelope that she's bad. Inside, the letter spreads chaotically to eight sides – I wish I didn't have to read it.

Dearest John

(just tired – NOT drunk!) I hope you enjoyed Mark Fry's 21st party ... Clare missed you in Box or at Colham, when she was in London – Malcolm P having visited her and taken her out to a wonderful (French) dinner ... followed by a visit to a 'wine bar'. Apparently he showed her London (they'd already had a carafe of red wine between two) and left her feeling lonely. Clare said she missed you v.much. You two are a great help to each other. Dear old Bill. I haven't recovered yet from his compliments about my paintings – not just remembered but very clearly so.

Dr R has just visited your Granny. He said Marjorie Incleton [her great friend] would not survive the shock etc, and that's what Frank thought. She's merely existing and would no doubt be happier to die. All her best friends and relations are dead.

I would so love to ring up Lise as I am Granny's unpaid 'home help'. She's welcome but there isn't much time left to write letters.

I realise my letter looks out of control but I'm OK, just overtired.

Frank and I saw *Women in Love* and *The Graduate* at the Wellesley. He preferred the latter. I think he's right. It was such a relief to laugh and tap one's feet after the overdone intensity of Ken Russell.

Since Dr R told Granny that MI was unlikely to survive the shocks at the age of 81, Granny has become almost hysterical. I'd better go and see her now. She was delighted with your letter.

So much love and good wishes to you from Mum, Frank, Sarah and Catherine.

Later.

I know I don't have an exactly calming effect on anyone but I am very hard pushed at the moment. It would be so nice if you could climb thro' a window or something on my birthday.

Mum xxx

ps. I'll be a painter yet.

She never puts 'good wishes'. She wants me to climb in through the window on her birthday like some knight in armour? Maybe she just means for something surprising to happen – in a way she's just bored stuck in Wellington. But I hate the way she still casually mentions my ex-girlfriend, wanting to ring her up on Granny's phone (Frank doesn't have a phone yet). I'm *not* with Lise, that's all over and done with. And she still hankers after 'Dear old Bill' Coldstream at the Slade, now her daughter's professor. To Mum it's all just yesterday: Yesterday's Papers, Yesterday's Man.

I did go to Mark's 21st in Box. Oh, I drank too much, smoked too much – there was some girl I was after who was only intent on being a cat, miaowing, rolling on the rug in front of the fire – until everything receded into the distance and I crawled off to sleep in a corner. Mum mentions Mark's because *she* went to that same house when I was young, when we lived just across the common. It's the same yearning as when she goes on about the 'wine bar', the *London* wine bar, that Clare's boyfriend has taken her to, with its wistful reference to the quantity of vino consumed. Mum, you're after some fiction of being married to Dad with everything hunky dory. Didn't you get divorced after the birth of your third child and then have a breakdown? Or did the breakdown come before the divorce? Mum, give up on all this rosy looking back.

Granny has come to live in Waterloo Road, next door to her only daughter, and they're proving they are the chalk and cheese they knew they were. Granny Betty suffered a stroke two winters ago in her bungalow in Rottingdean. She had been alone there, for several years, since the death of dear Peter, her second husband. Putting up a picture over the mantelpiece, she fell. She lay on the floor, holding on to the radiator for eleven hours. Her hand on that radiator was what saved her, she said. She was still hanging on in the bungalow when Frank and Mum went to see her and decided that the only real option was for her to come and live with them. Frank's mother hadn't survived long after her stroke and he expected it would be the same with Betty, though as it turned out she would live another six years, more or less on top of them. So they moved her to the 'tropical' West Country, where it rained all the time and the humidity gave her rheumatism, and she hated it from the start. How she resented it, complained, longed to get back home to Sussex. At first she lived upstairs in Clare's old bedroom, her belongings piled up around her – a Miss Haversham in bed in the midst of it all, hair in a horrible plastic cap, teeth in a glass beside her. Her furniture arrived from Rottingdean and filled up the downstairs back room. She had everyone at her beck and call. Of course it was intolerable for the five people already living there. Then, after four months, the ground-floor flat next door miraculously fell vacant and she was moved in there. Frank had a buzzer installed through the party wall to our sitting room – and she used it. Mum now had a job after all, and full time. Keeping a constant eye on her mother should have been good for her, and in some ways it probably was, but it was also a great strain. The strain that had once lived far away in Sussex, and then unbearably in the bedroom next to hers, was now alive and better and vigorously complaining next door at 69A.

I wonder about my other granny, so different. So classy.

Helen may be in her autumn Sloane Square hotel right now, just a short walk from Harrods, but I don't think of contacting her and dropping in again for tea. I don't go there again, though my sisters do. So I never did see Granny Helen again. She died quite suddenly a few years later.

Over Christmas at Colham I talk about my future with my father. He comes up with something more about Olivier. There had always been this family connection with his mother, from her stage days, and when he was at school Dad wrote to him asking if he should take up acting as a profession, and Olivier wrote back: No! Later, when he was stationed in India at the end of the war, he saw him on stage in Calcutta entertaining the troops. Then, back to England, demobbed, he heard the actor was setting off for a tour of Australia and he tried again, asked if he could join the tour. 'The answer was an unequivocal no. So I became a painter instead,' says Dad, chomping on his pipe.

We talk about what I'm going to do, now I've got away from London, out of Turnpike Lane. We light our pipes, his straight and plain, mine currently a curved Petersen briar. He paces the sitting room, while I look into the log fire. I want to go back to art school, but somewhere new. Fine Art not History of Art. I just want to paint. 'How about Falmouth? They have a tradition of figurative painting there.' It's far away, the very opposite of London, and immediately appealing. He rings Francis Hewlett, whom he knew at the Slade, and explains my predicament. Might I be able to transfer from Reading to Falmouth, as it were. I accept my father's intervention, the element of nepotism, gratefully, and get an interview.

I go down on the train a couple of weeks later. Oh evocative journey, entering Cornwall, stopping at all the stations: Liskeard, Lostwithiel, St Austell, Bodmin Parkway, Truro. Change at Truro for Falmouth. It's actually the first time I've been to Cornwall.

Despite living almost all of my twenty years in Wiltshire, Dorset and Somerset, I've never been further west than Dartmoor; I haven't crossed the Tamar. How warm it is down there for January, and wet. Alighting at the small empty platform of the Dell, I relish the mildness, the kindness of the air. Walking the rain-drenched streets, climbing the hill to the art school with a great vista of the harbour below, the gardens apparently full of exotic palms, it feels a million miles from Reading. It looks a great place to be.

The interview seems to go well, and I'm surprised to be rejected on the spot. They suggest that I try again, through the usual channels. Get some work in my portfolio and come back in May. I have four months, I think, as the train winds its way back through the wooded Cornish valleys. I'll paint hard and make a portfolio that will get me into Falmouth. But where can I live to do that?

10. A Colham winter

Dad offers me Colham until the end of March. They will be in their new house in Reading this term. Since Francesca's birth they have been spending more time at his place of work and less in the country. 'You can look after the place and the cat. We'll come to visit occasionally, if that's all right with you!' he banters.

It's a considerable gesture on his part – I've never stayed there on my own before. Colham has always been only our holiday home. It's where my sisters and I *visit*. But I'm certain about going to Cornwall and he probably senses that. I haven't been so sure and determined since I left home to live with Lise in Bristol three years ago. He wants to help and I'm only too glad to take up his offer to live and paint at Colham for the rest of the winter. Of course I'll look after the place! Not only the house, but also his studio. For he has turned his pictures to the wall and given me the run of the studio 'for three months only'. I'll be sleeping in there with a camp bed in the corner.

'Don't get lonely,' Catherine H says, as they drive away up the track, and I don't believe I will. Looking round at the damp grey winter valley I'm sure I will be happy in my solitude.

I have the house, the valley, to myself. Lettie, their short-haired grey cat with startling orange eyes, is my companion. The postman comes down the track to deliver my mail. There's a baker, grocer and post office in the village. There's a freezer and cupboard of food. But I won't cook much. Not for one. Just plenty of bacon and egg, and the Italian version: spaghetti alla carbonara. The old portable black and white television is in the corner if I need it. I pick up my bird diary of the previous summer, unopened during the three months in London: *Twilight at the studio window as it all becomes dark and rich in silence … Robins singing everywhere … Moorhens talking to each other. Had to kill a starling Lettie brought in at midnight.*

I settle in, go for walks around the valley I know so well. I want to know it better, everything about it. I follow the river upstream to its source beyond the village and downstream to the A4. I watch the winter slowly turn, the buds thicken, the days lengthen.

And I set about making as many images as I can. I grab all the hours of daylight, and work on into the twilight, the best time, when getting the thing down on paper before the light goes is most urgent. When it's finally too dark I take advantage of the powerful spotlights in the studio and work into the night. I puff away on my pipe, which becomes my constant painting companion. You could say I live in a cloud of smoke.

What am I doing in all this drawing and painting? I hardly know. I just throw myself into a stream of work on paper, canvas and board, with pencil, ink, watercolour, acrylic, collage. I paint interiors of the house, and what I can see of the valley through the windows; sometimes it's dry enough to work outside, but most of the time I stay in. There's enough inside to keep me going for three months.

I love the plain, austere interior of my father's house. Wood, plaster, stone. White walls. No carpets, not even curtains. The floors are of dark-polished wood, with a little rush matting in the sitting room; the main windows have folding wooden shutters, the rest are bare. The sparse furniture tends to be 'monumental'. There are one or two sculptures – the Towers Bra on top of the stripped cupboard – but almost nothing on the walls. A Victorian case of butterflies up on the wall but no paintings. None of *his* paintings. 'Not going to spoil the place with my efforts,' blusters Dad. This might all seem rather spartan and distinctly lacking in creature comforts but it isn't. The house is warm and dry with the recently installed central heating. It's just uncluttered, simple, with no concession to prettiness. There are no knick-knacks –

how different from my mother's. How calming.

I focus on these elements of the house: the massive walls, white plaster curves, plain winding staircase, ancient beams; dark wood, small windows, that cavernous fireplace. And a few select objects that are closer to my father: a shiny brass bedpost, the wheel-back armchair, the scrubbed kitchen sideboard, a blue bottle placed just so on the windowsill, some golden daffs in a white jug. I look out of the windows to the valley beyond – the hill across the river, three pines at the top; bend of the river by the heron oak (where several herons roost every night) – and add some of the exterior to the interior elements. If this all sounds rather lofty, it's only an *aim*. The actual work is more a case of putting everything down on the paper, of suck it and see.

Sometimes I go up to the village in the evening, ensconce myself in the White Hart Inn with a book, stumble home through the fields in the gloaming. In my diary I write: *Living at Colham my time is divided perfectly between painting, music, birdwatching, reading and housework.* Indeed, it's very different from my autumn in London. On painting I enter: *Work at the moment: large abstract of shape and colour after Dad but it doesn't matter; small, detailed, semi-naturalistic ones – better.*

There's a power cut one day from 3 p.m. to midnight and the track is all vans and men working by torchlight – a JCB has cut through a major cable and the whole village has been blacked out. *Romantic candle and fire evening with Lettie the cat!*

A couple of days later in a storm, seven trees are blown down in the valley, including two huge elms *torn out by the roots, which reach up at least twelve feet tall.*

An inch of snow in the morning but it melted away quickly, I note with regret.

Gigantic yellow moon peeps over the hill at dusk; gets smaller as it rises.

I do some detective work on a badger sett in the wood above the heron tree, sift through the fresh bedding outside it, find shredded pine cones and fresh grubbings with claw marks in the earth.

I stalk a buzzard in a tree for half an hour, then watch it soar, hang with wings folded, drop like a stone on its prey.

Then I go back to listen to records: Bach's *Orchestral Suites*, Spanish harp music, a Julian Bream guitar recital with Ravel's exquisite *Pavane pour une infante défunte*.

Upstairs in the studio I have my new Philips cassette recorder and a small collection of the new cassette tapes. It was bought on Frank's recommendation while I was living in London. I'm proud of this little machine, which I regard as 'high tech'. It was a *Which?* Best Buy and to get it I trekked out to the first Comet shop, then a modest electrical goods outlet on the Finchley Road. We've always had *Which?* at home. Frank was an early subscriber: 'It's the only non-advertising and therefore unbiased magazine.' We grew up with their Best Buys, from toasters to irons to transistor radios to washing powders ('Square Deal Surf') and my 'Beirette II', a simple fixed lens 35mm camera, which replaced my first Box Brownie.

I doggedly pursue a routine of exercises and scales for classical guitar, sitting correctly with my left foot up on a stool, guitar wedged between my legs. To progress I must learn to read music. I get a manuscript book into which I copy scores by hand – *Prelude No* 1 by Villa-Lobos. I make photocopies when I can and stick them in – Ravel's *Pavane*. Between painting sessions and in the evening I relax with Dylan and Cohen and Simon and Garfunkel songs. The chords and lyrics are written out at the back of my 'classical' book. I strum, hum, whistle and sing, sometimes yell them through the uncurtained windows into the night.

My father comes down for his birthday weekend, and we

make a day trip to Slimbridge. Catherine H is keen on birds too; music and birds are the touchstones of my friendship with my stepmother, who is still a fairly new stepmother to me. This is my second visit to Slimbridge, the first having been in my young teens soon after it opened, when I ran everywhere, thrilled to bits. I find the place as enchanting as ever, especially the wild swan viewing room with its great plate-glass window and an exhibition of Peter Scott's watercolours showing that every wild Bewick's and Whooper swan has a different and diagnostic pattern to its bill. When we leave for Slimbridge in the morning after a night of heavy rain, the river is within two feet of flooding the house. On our return in the evening it's swilling outside the back door. A glint of water is visible through the cracks in the dining room floor. In 1968 the house was flooded – the river ran right through it – and when we came for our summer holidays there was a two-foot high tide mark around the walls and a lot of ruined books. Now we set to, Dad, Catherine H and I, to avoid another disaster. Dad is in bombastic military mood, blustering like his father. In military fashion he deploys his troops to raise the cooker off the floor, take up the rush matting, balance the sofa precariously between four chairs. We go up to bed uneasily. But next day it stops and the water level slowly goes down. I watch the swollen river from the window: a dabchick battling the current, a plump of moorhens in the flooded fields, two herons back on their tree.

They go back to Reading. It's too wet to work out. I stoke up my pipe and choose a view from a window. *Magpies and crows have attacked the putty on the windows again*, I note. We don't know why they do this – Dad says it's the birds attacking us; it's like his belief that peacock feathers in the house bring bad luck.

Andrew comes down from the farm on his tractor. He's a year older than me and seems more. He drives the tractor everywhere, hunting for scrap metal he can turn into cash, and he finds plenty. Not the small-time stuff we turn up around the outhouse and garden but great hunks and slabs of rusty iron from the fields and barns and cowsheds; he collects it by the ton. He has just lost, without regret, his £100 wager with his mother about not smoking a cigarette before the age of twenty-one, which she believed would at least have given him a chance to save himself from the evils of tobacco addiction. She herself is a lifelong heavy smoker and it will kill her in the end; she'll get emphysema in thirty years time and with the agony of it, the hopelessness, take her own life. But now Andrew thinks nothing of losing the bet with his mother: he wants to smoke, as we all do. He's a combative man; I've played him many times at squash in my teens and never won. One day he brings me an anti-EEC petition to sign, arguing vehemently against the disastrous centralisation of power and choking bureaucracy that the Common Market will bring upon everyone. I'm not at all sure about this. My instinct always is to be with Europe.

Andrew keeps me up with the news: Heath embroiled with the miners; a 50 mph limit on motorways to conserve fuel; Britain on a three-day week. This doesn't seem a such bad thing to me at all. Most people would surely be happier working three days and spending the rest of the time following their interests. Though I'm happy with my own current seven-day week and wouldn't want to reduce that at all. Time is running on and the work ahead seems infinite: the more you do, the more is to be done.

A likeable Swiss friend of Andrew's comes down from the farm. Rudi sits on the floor in the studio for an hour looking at my pictures while I work, daydreaming, he says. When he gets back to Switzerland, he will go to prison for refusing the draft. It will give him plenty of time to read and write, he says. On his last night, Andrew and I go up to the pub with the philosophical Swiss and get plastered.

The postman bumps down the track, bringing pale blue envelopes from Kent. They are for Dad and of course I know who they are from. The very same arrive at home, and have done as far back as I can remember; letters from our first stepmother, Corinne, sometimes for Mum, sometimes for us children too. They are scarily mad. Corinne is in a hospice in Whitstable, Kent. She has been there for years but there has never been a chance of going to see her. Dad never talks about her – all that's in the past and somehow taboo. Except that these letters keep arriving. I put them in his pile of mail. Will they be mentioned at all when he comes down at the weekend? He has a new family now, a new life, and Corinne, like my mother, was his old one.

Corinne was an artist too, a sculptor. She was a sculpture student at Corsham (Bath Academy of Art) where Dad taught. Talented. Won a prize for her sculpture *Standing Figure*. There's a clipping from the *Western Daily Press* at home, another of Granny's finds. The photograph I have of this sculpture shows an amazing piece of work, a larger than life plaster figure, with Corinne working at it in a man's shirt too big for her, in her socks, plaster-splattered, applying the wet plaster with her hands with an expression of great concentration. I knew Corinne when I was five. She was my mother when my own mum disappeared. Then *she* disappeared back to her home in Whitstable. She never came here to Colham, never saw this wonderful place.

What happened to her? And do I still have a young half-sister, Amanda? I only ever saw her once, one Christmas when she was six months old. She was lying in a tinselled crib inside Dad's igloo tent in their house at Bath, a tableau that showed my father at his most theatrical, and a wonderful creation it was.

There are letters from Mum and Frank too. Mum's letters often seem to be on the edge like Corinne's, but she isn't too bad at the moment. She's trying to be 'on the level'. The trouble is, however hard she tries you can't help reading between the lines.

Frank writes his regular letters. I've always had letters from Frank. He has been writing reassuringly to me ever since I was seven at boarding school. Whenever I was away from home for any length of time, he would write. My sisters got them too – he wrote a lot of letters – though being younger (and not at boarding school), they only received theirs later on. Clare will be getting them at the Slade now. Frank's letters bring the real news from home. They tell you just what's going on, often quite bluntly. They tell you about Mum and don't pussyfoot around.

23.1.74

Dear John,

Good news. I think the worst is over with Mum and she is on an upward gradient. She is lucky not to have landed in hospital and the police court. I know all about the shoplifting as well now and some you don't know. Last week she pinched two bottles of whisky – one on Wednesday when we went to Taunton and one straight after seeing her psychiatrist. She took something from Chapmans after seeing you off on Saturday. All incredible and extremely lucky. We should have had front page of the *Wellington Weekly*, a court case and Tone Vale [psychiatric hospital] I'm sure. So it was lucky I came across that half bottle of brandy and got tough with her.

We are having nothing to drink in the house at all for a month or so and there is a padlock on the cellar door. She already seems a reformed character, friendly and helpful. So a better visit next time! Clare is coming tomorrow for a weekend. Is all well with you? Let's hear what is going on. Some good paintings coming along, I'm sure.

I went round the town last Saturday and paid off all Mum's debts – about £25, but I think that is all.

All good wishes, Frank.

31.1.74
Dear John,
I hope the river isn't rising too much where you are. We've lost 6 milk bottles (smashed) in the last two windy nights. The latest accusation from Granny is that she hid her diamond and sapphire engagement ring from my father in the cactus with red fruit. As far as I remember that cactus has never been in her house, though I may have put it down for a few mins on my way back from the W.I. She has lost and found with Frank's help her cultured pearls again ... Please write to Clare at the Slade as our letters sent to previous addresses have not been forwarded so far. She is safe in her new room now. Bill Coldstream has got 'The Slade' badly and evidently only remarried in order to have a woman to take to social functions whom he is proud to display. Love from a reformed and struggling Mum.

From Frank again:

... Mum's hand is healing but she has to go to East Reach [hospital] on Thursday about it. On the same day she is seeing an 'alcoholic counsellor' [sic] about her problem. Dr. Bradfield suggested this. So when you next come home lock up your money and don't bring any drink ... We saw *Last Tango in Paris* at the Wellesley on Thursday but though I'm glad I saw it I didn't think it very good ... I found myself mentally going over a chess game I had played earlier in the day several times during the film. Still, it was an evening out.

Thanks for your letter. Write again! Yrs Frank.

And Mum next day:

Thank you for your letter – it gave me the giggles. Sarah and Catherine have them most of the time, especially Sarah. She looks about 13 now and v. sweet in her patchwork navy and white dress, like a child in *Alias Smith and Jones*. Puts herself to bed, washes up, etc, etc, due to Catherine making her!

I am going (voluntarily) to see a counsellor on Alcoholism next week after yet another visit to East Reach.

Frank and I saw *Last Tango in Paris* last night at the Wellesley, v.g. but MB did seem to have rather a one-track mind. He didn't seem up to doing even as little in life as I do.

Night night. Love Mum.

At least she can laugh at herself. The difference in their views on *Last Tango* are pretty much the differences between them. But the 'hand healing' in Frank's letter, which Mum herself doesn't mention, refers to a severe cut on her wrist from when she punched through the glass of Granny's front door after her mother had locked her out. The glass sliced close to the artery. Blood everywhere. Ambulance. I'd like to think Granny was up to the situation, as she was once a fully-trained nurse, but more likely she cowered in bed until the ambulance came, enraged and helpless at another attack by her daughter. This always happened when Mum 'got bad', or you could say when Frank effectively sealed off other sources of cash to buy liquor and Granny's purse became a bottomless pot to be worked over with all the guile of the addict.

Who staunched the blood? Put on the tourniquet? If it wasn't Granny, I suppose it would have been Frank. The only reference Mum makes is 'yet another visit to the hospital'. The cut does take a long time to heal and will be troublesome for years. Perhaps she is ashamed this time. Perhaps the whole sorry event has really disturbed her; she has seen herself step too far, scare her poor mother out of her wits. There's such a destructive power in Mum. Everything is bottled up and sometimes it has to explode. Frank just says she's an alcoholic and tries to stem all sources of booze – again and again he tries but she always finds a way round. *Why* she is an alcoholic, no one ever seems to ask.

Catherine writes to me too. She's singing 'Bushes and Briars' from the film *Far from the Madding Crowd* for her music exam, is still deciding which A levels to do at the Tech. She has talked to someone helpful there who actually believes that it's a good idea to go to college, unlike at her school. From her secondary modern she's very conscious of elder brother and sister going to university and art school and is struggling to match them (she will in fact end up going to the Slade too). She's seeking reassurance from me – I don't know how helpful I am. We have this close bond that manifests itself in a shared sense of humour. How easily I can make her laugh with a Peter Cook or Frankie Howerd impression. I can do the 'eyebrow thing' – raise my crooked right eyebrow quizzically, a trait we have both inherited from our father – and guarantee to get her laughing. Then she speaks about Mum:

> ... Mum has been struggling to copy a Cézanne still life – it is very painful to see her sometimes. I don't know if you have ever felt like I do about her, but sometimes when she is so depressed and tries to comfort herself by drinking and eating – always in secret as though she is hunted – it is heart-breaking. Frank thinks she has stopped drinking and is giving her more money, but I know she hasn't. It is as though there is nothing left in life for her and she has very little pleasure, always escaping by going out or to bed and always being grumbled at and told off – it's awful.

I'm impressed by my sister's understanding, and her sympathy. How similar, really, her thoughts on Mum are to my own. Below the scoffing exterior, the critical angry son, there is so much else I feel about my mother.

I invite De Gruyter and Lise down from Reading for the day. Why do I do that? Why do I want my ex and her partner to visit me at Colham? I'm just so proud of living here, working at my painting. I want to show them my domain. I'm over my jealousy – they are married now – and would like to be friends, on an equal footing. Lise always loved it here at Colham. They seem happy enough to come.

Late morning there's a call from the top of the hill. Lise is waving by the stile. They'll have parked up there on the road. I climb the steep hill and give them a tour of the valley. We walk round the upper end, as far as derelict Nettleton Mill, which we decide to buy and turn into an artist's community, living self-sufficiently, using the old mill for power – all living together, note. I will continue to do paintings of the valley and sell them in local galleries. I rabbit on, full of optimism, high on showing them round my domain. We circle round to the village for lunch in the White Hart.

It was last summer they got married – in Paris. An amazing coincidence, they were in Paris, living and working at Shakespeare & Co. bookshop, when I passed through. Maybe that time I was sleeping on Sylvie's floor I could have gone to their wedding. There are grumbles about the Art Department. Dee is still getting flak for her figurative work. Terry Frost's comment on her etchings was that they'd be nice to show her mother. While her least favourite visiting lecturer from London suggested during a tutorial, while brandishing a screwdriver, that what she really needed was a good screw. Through Dee's tears of anguish, her rage at the injustice of it, De Gruyter and Lise are providing support, championing her work.

We go back to the house, where I put Bach on the record player for them, and De Gruyter and I both draw portraits of Lise sitting bolt upright in the wheel-back armchair. Diary: *Remarkably dissimilar portraits, one hard and one soft, neither any good.* I also take a photograph of Lise in the wheel-back, for a painting I will never do. I note an evening of reading and music and cooking, and *regrettably a few private tears, which I'm very glad I concealed, though I think Lise knew.* They leave and I give my best to the guitar before going to bed, playing for Lise as she speeds away up the M4 to Reading. I muse about living without a wife, how you could be stronger, get more done on your own if you could stand the loneliness: *Be a lifelong bachelor but keep the mysterious lady of dreams. I'm still only twenty, seem to have been that age for years.*

Dutch Elm Disease has reached the valley and many elms are being felled this winter. The air fills with the roar of chainsaws. Nine full grown trees come down along the track in a single morning. Two days later: *25 elms felled in the valley but, oddly, it hasn't made much difference to the views.* While they are cutting, I stay indoors on a mammoth painting session of 15 hours until 3 a.m. I'm working on a series of trees, based on what I can see from the studio window, fragmenting them in a cubist way; I paint thinly in acrylics which are transparent and easily overlaid, as well as drying quickly. I know I'm very much imitating my father in this.

There's a Saturday shoot, which I hate. Shooting in the countryside has always upset me, even hearing it while on a walk. It goes back to early childhood and Bob, the English master-cum-gamekeeper at my boarding school, who practically brought his smoking twelve-bore into the classroom, who kept a grisly larder of the birds and animals he had shot, crow to pigeon, stoat to rabbit, like the cruel gamekeepers in books. What gets me by the throat is these men swinging their haul of pheasants and mallards by the neck and chucking them into the boots of their Daimlers. No different from what my grandfather did, which was probably where I first saw this utter contempt for wild creatures. At Colham I got into trouble as a teenager for pulling up all the marker sticks where the hunters are to stand, and I don't feel any different about it now.

I continue to note what I see: the date of the first primrose and wild daffodil; the first butterfly, a brimstone; first summer migrant, a chiffchaff. I still do this. It punctuates the year. And I think about taking a degree in ecology with the Open University. Living here quietly at Colham I would be able to do that as well as paint. I could express my love for nature through science *and* art, I think, as I wander about the valley poking into its nooks and crannies.

The end looms, 30 March, and I go into overdrive. There now seem to be infinite paintings I haven't done. I lay a lot of half finished things out on the studio floor, work on them in a circular way as I've seen my father do – the first one is dry when you come back to it. I do a painting of Lettie, sitting on the back of the sofa, looking with the viewer through to the dining room – perhaps more my mother's influence here; she used to be a great painter of cats. I struggle to get the light from the small windows reflecting on the polished wood of the floor and table, on the tops of the bentwood chairs, and then on Lettie's silver-grey fur. It's a slight picture, I think, but Mum will later claim it and put it up in the sitting room at Waterloo Road, where it remains to this day.

Then I do one of my best drawings. On a bright March day I take my board up the hill, heading for a place at the end of the valley that I've had my eye on for some time. The marsh marigolds are shining in the mill ditch, there are sunny celandine faces everywhere, dog violets on the mossy slope. Over a wall, under barbed wire, across the muddy footpath. I climb higher, reach the dry tussocky grass, and sit with the board on my knees. The whole valley lies below me: looping river through the bare winter trees, heron tree at the centre, steep tobogganing slope and Colham Wood. The sun comes out. It grows beautifully warm. I sit there so still I become part of the landscape. Rabbits come out. Birds sing like mad in the blackthorn, carry on with their chasing, chattering and diving. I work rapidly in charcoal, no rubbing out, not giving it much thought; feeling it's right, that it's all clicking into place. When I've lugged my drawing back to the house and stepped back from it, I know this is the best I can do.

A few years ago, I found this same drawing again, in my old pre-art school portfolio under a bed; it seemed worthy of a frame and a place in our house. And then, just recently, my father saw it. He was drawn towards it, I could see, even as we sat talking. After a while he asked if it was Colham valley, on the high path to the village. Yes, he remembered the view well. Hadn't I spent some time at Colham once, painting on my own? He stroked his beard, trying to remember. Then he said that it was a very fine drawing. Nearly forty years later – a marriage, a family, a career – this unsolicited praise from my father still carried power.

Suddenly it's the last evening and alas how little I've done. Looking through the windows, stepping outside to look at the river and weir, I keep seeing unpainted paintings. But my time is up. Dad is back in the house and reclaiming his studio. I pack up my things portfolio, quite a fat portfolio, and go back to Wellington, from *the incredible calm of Colham to the chaos of Wellington*. I'm eternally grateful to my father for giving me this opportunity. I only wish it had been longer, a full turn of the year.

There's a little Colham ps. A week later I'm back there in another hat: elder brother with two sisters come for Dad's spring holiday. The weather is sultry. *Rain: the valley full of rich earthy smells and a dense background of birdsong. Kingfisher and dipper glimpsed,* I record fondly. But we don't stay in our Wiltshire valley. They've rented a cottage in Kirkby Malham (Catherine H is a Yorkshire lass) for a week – I must have my twenty-first birthday there but have no memory or record of it. We spend most of the week in bed with a gastric bug. Everyone goes down with it, there's vomiting galore. On the last day, I note, we are well enough to visit Gordale Scar, subject of a famous Turner watercolour in the Tate; the moors are full of the wild mournful calls of curlews, the piping of redshanks come there to nest. Returning to Colham – why did we ever go away? – I feel how perfect it all is: *Everything has grown up a lot in the last week ... the valley lush and green ... willow warblers singing everywhere ... the best month of May approaching.*

But we're leaving Colham, we all are. The house has been let for a year to the Stringers, some artist friends of Dad's. We're packing up and clearing out.

The name 'Stringer' triggers a memory of a summer party with the Hopes in Box. We'd been going to the Hopes to play cricket on their lawn for years; the Frys, who lived nearby, came too; what began as a cricket match would segue into a barbecue and party. Joe Hope was a keen cricketer who played for Box village team, and to us seemed brilliant. Of course we knew he was playing down to us, on his titchy home lawn with a tennis ball, but he never showed it. Forty, paunchy, grinning ferociously, Joe bowled his deadly spinners at me and Mark, at his sons and my sisters, even his toddler daughter, building up the spirit of competition in us. There was a large greenhouse about ten yards behind the bowler's arm and there was a forfeit for any ball that was hit anywhere *near* his greenhouse; we had smashed a few a panes over the years, even Joe when he overdid it. It was an exciting and hot afternoon. Drinks were brought out towards the end, 'pop' for us, alcohol for the adults, and cricket morphed into something else; we teenagers tucked into the free booze. On this occasion the Stringers and the Hodgkins came. Music blared through open windows onto the lawn. The grown-ups got up and danced, and got off with each other. Mr H danced with Mrs S, while her husband looked on, miserably, we thought, from the 'children's table'; Dad went off with the host. Mark and I swigged our drinks and watched. There were no girls of our age; we weren't going to dance with our sisters. The couples on the lawn were smooching now, holding tight, mouths glued together in kisses lasting minutes. After a while Dad and his new friend slipped back from the bottom of the garden. It was an artists' party.

We are packing up Colham for the Stringers. A few more days and we'll be losing it for a year or more. I feel the loss acutely after my three-month residency as I gather together the last of my possessions, the little treasures found on all those childhood holidays – a few more fossils from the ploughed fields and limestone walls, Roman pottery fragments from my archaeology on Truckle Hill, butterflies from my days as a lepidopterist, birds' egg fragments, feathers, a wren's nest, the odd exotic item such as a sawfish jaw Dad once gave me – to take to my room at Waterloo Road, which will again be my home for the summer. But I have a second interview at Falmouth School of Art in a fortnight.

11. Summer at Mum's

This time I get in. I have a place at Falmouth in the autumn. The gap has been filled again. I hang around Wellington for most of the summer. It is not a good summer at Waterloo Road. Clare has disappeared up to London. Catherine is at the Taunton Tech and often away staying with friends. Little Sarah is at school. Frank is at school. And Mum is a shadow in her bedroom, only seeming to emerge in belligerence. I wish I could find something positive to say about her here, but there is only an insistent memory of one of her drink-fuelled adventures this summer – in a moment.

Broke after my three months in the country, I go up to the labour exchange and get a job in Debenham's Post Room in Taunton. I'll be putting letters in pigeon holes. Exciting work. Though in my case I know it's temporary, and my mind can be elsewhere. Now that I know I'm going back to college, I'm no longer condemned to a dogsbody job like this for the rest of my life; I feel sorry for these guys who are. Still, it's a long office day, with an hour's travel each way, and it grinds me down. My bird diary of the Colham winter dries up: the only entries for several months are for a grey wagtail seen from the office window and the large numbers of mallards with young waddling round Taunton town centre; they have special duck road signs. At home I go for an evening walk to Nynehead Hollow on the edge of town tracking a nightingale reported in the local paper, but don't find it. I still haven't heard a nightingale in England. It's a lonely time, spiritless – all the comforts of home but not appreciating them, hating being there. There are probably one or two people from school still around but I make no effort to contact them.

I must do some painting before the start of term, continue from where I left off at Colham, hopefully keep up the momentum.

I try a still life, based partly on Braque's *Guéridon* series which I've been admiring in a little Penguin monograph: the old spinet in the sitting room, with Mum's antique mirror, her vase of dried seedheads and honesty flowers and a case of stuffed birds recently given to her (or us) by her mother; the 'guéridon', a three-legged black *papier maché* table in the bay window, is in the reflection. I tip the perspective to flatten the picture plane, make it facetted and Cubist; imitate Braque's subdued palette, his soft warm greys. I do two of these sketchy paintings in acrylic. Mum likes them, and I appreciate her comments in a moment of calm. Whatever else she is or isn't, I respect her artistic eye – at least she can still give me this. The pictures are abandoned quite early on and left at home, gummed on the drawing board. Later, when I need the drawing board, they are torn off and stowed among my youthful work for the next thirty-two years, until they have a fortunate resurrection. A friend – it's Martin from Reading Fine Art class of 1971 – picks them out as the cover for my book of poems, *Eggshell: A Decorator's Notes*.

I also pursue the idea of doing an ecology degree with the Open University in tandem with a fine art degree – I don't want to risk all my eggs in one art basket. But when the introductory package arrives from the OU, I find it difficult. Not having done science to A level, I have to catch up, and I'm suddenly thrown into a series of, to me, weird physics-and-chemistry-at-home experiments. Frank, scientifically inclined and ever the enthusiast, helps me with these improvisations. Thus we test magnetism, Boyle's law, whatever, with an assortment of culinary equipment rigged up on the kitchen table. This is just the kind of thing Frank likes and we get on fine doing the experiments. But something in my head still refuses to grapple with the logic and rigour of science, its tedious charts and graphs, as it always has. I will take the course down to Falmouth with me and persevere with it through the first term, but there I find I can't or won't play these science games myself – I really can't be bothered to set up all this lab stuff in the communal kitchen.

Frank introduces me to Edward de Bono's *Lateral Thinking*, another challenge. Here's a bit of his five-day course in thinking: *Day 2. Find whether it's possible to construct a platform on top of four milk bottles, using only four kitchen knives. The platform must be strong enough to support a full glass of water between the bottles, which must be positioned slightly more than a knife length apart. Only the four knives can be used, and no part of them may touch the ground.* It is possible, delightfully achievable after all, and actually I dearly want to 'think laterally' like this – it seems to me this has much to do with what art and poetry is about. But, like art, I discover, it can't be forced; it needs to be approached at an angle, intuition is involved. Working on de Bono's problems, I watch my mind obstinately sticking to straighter lines than it should, getting itself trapped on the hamster's treadmill and refusing to step outside. I think I can't write poetry for the same reasons, only gushes of feeling, and all that I keep to myself.

I'm still getting over Lise. It's taking a long time. Eighteen months since we broke up, the reactive flings have come and gone, and I have found no one to replace her. Her mother writes in reply to what must have been a miserable missive from me: 'What are friends for?' she says kindly and invites me (vaguely) to visit her in Oxford. She has closed the coffee shop in Wellington and gone to where her heart lies. She talks about my mother a bit, how the psychiatrists haven't been much use to her, how psychiatrists with their bucketloads of drugs don't help anyone. It's a sympathetic letter and touching to receive so long after I've 'left' her family, but I also feel it's her vindication in the end; she was never happy about my relationship with her daughter from the start. I don't want to phone her – that would be just be pointlessly hanging on. No, I'm not going to phone her. (I won't ever see her again.) I'll stay sad in my old childhood room instead. In my loss, frustration and anger, and surely confusion about my own mother, I sing along with David Bowie's 'Rebel Rebel' on the radio. I love the rhyme about getting your mother in a whirl, not sure if you're a boy or a girl. I doubt it would put my mother in a whirl, though. She's okay at least with boys being girls and girls being boys. 'Seen it all,' she says airily of her time at art school. When Clare comes home for a weekend, we go to a dance at the local rugby club. We bop to Bowie – *he's OUTRAGEOUS* – under the bright canteen lights and she suddenly laughs at my stuck-out 'Elvis' jaw. But Clare this is how you do it these days: pursed lips, rockstar pout, defiant jaw; thumb in the loop of your jeans and a shake of your shaggy head. She's probably laughing too from embarrassment at being out with her brother.

But our mum is behaving badly at home this summer. She's nearly at her worst. I document one of her bad days: 'Mum: A Day in the Life, July 1974', after John Lennon, after a Solzhenitsyn novella I've just read, *One Day in the Life of Ivan Denisovich*, a devastating little tale of the futility of human endeavour.

> I was up at nine, early. There was a note from Mum to make the lunch while she was in Taunton seeing Dr Bradfield. I carried on carpenting a wooden box for my oil pastels and forgot the time; Sarah and Catherine arrived home for lunch, they were both in high spirits. We put together some lunch and then Mum arrived back, also in a good mood, as she usually is after seeing her psychiatrist. She told us she was going to get a job, part-time, no more drinking. We didn't believe her; she's never had a job. Then she went out.
>
> At four, with Sarah already back from school and watching Playschool, Mum came in
>
> with her wild battered look – totally sloshed. She went

straight up to bed before Frank got in. Radio 1 blared from the bedroom. She told Frank she was ill and he believed her. Something was going to happen, we were sure of it. The house remained peaceful while Frank got on and cooked the supper. Mum was called and came down all meek and mild. When I took Granny her supper next door, she was hostile towards her 'thieving daughter'; she says Mum came in this morning and stole some money. Then Frank found a three-quarters empty bottle of Scotch in a shopping basket by the dustbin. There was a furious argument which ended with Mum slamming off out. Frank went round to Granny's to tell her to lock up her cash, and discovered that Mum had indeed taken £5 this morning, having persuaded her to give it to me as a leaving present. He found empties stashed there too. Granny is absolutely terrified of Mum at the moment and isn't going to let her into the flat any more. It was only Tuesday and Mum had spent the entire week's housekeeping, and my £5, on booze. And now she was out somewhere in the town.

The doorbell rang. It was Finn, the Vice-head from school, bringing Mum home. Vice-head, he's called; he's in charge of my mother's vices. She'd come knocking on his door, begging for cash (though he didn't actually say this). It was so ridiculous, him asking if Mum was all right, when everyone could see she was completely off her head. Frank thanked Finn – how awful he must have felt – and tried to appease Mum. He said he was glad she had come back. He gets so scared when Mum's like this. She's beyond his control, anything might happen.

'I'm not staying,' she said out loud to everyone. 'Been offered £2.50 a time at the chip shop. You can't even keep it up.'

It was terribly embarrassing.

Mum put Sarah to bed. The one job she had to do every night, and she did it. Then raged around the house shouting at everyone. She pursued us – me, Catherine, Frank – from room to room, but left the room if we spoke back at her. She was like a spoilt kid, pathetic, dreadful, we said. But beyond our embarrassment and shame, we were deeply worried. Frank was now on the phone to Dr Richardson. He came into the sitting room where we were waiting and announced Mum was certifiable and that a breakdown was probably coming on. Mum had been listening too. She came in and stood at the door, then went quietly up to bed.

Not only Mum. Granny Betty is also causing a rumpus next door now. I note:

Sunday morning. Ring at the door at 1.30 a.m. – a sergeant and two constables with Granny. They had found her wandering in the town, recognised her and brought her back home. They were worried and said she should be in hospital. Granny was in good spirits and seemed to think it was a game, that she had been rather clever. Her door was open and chairs etc had been dragged down the path as though she was moving house.

Granny Betty's flat at 69A is now chockablock. Everything from Rottingdean has arrived and been crammed in. Now she spends her time hunting for 'lost' things, things put in a safe place. The diamond engagement ring from Peter, her big sparkler, the one she said she hid in the cactus and Mum went off with, occupies acres of time. When she isn't hunting for the Ring, she's busy getting her papers in a muddle – all the saved letters, policies, statements, bills … But not always. Sometimes she's given up on all that and is to be found sitting quietly, bolstered by pillows in her high bed, reading. Her *Express*, her thrillers, or today, gratifyingly, the Penguin *War and Peace* I gave her for her birthday.

I've brought her supper round on a tray. Placed the tray on the brick wall between our two front gardens and vaulted it. You can go out the gate and along the pavement and in Granny's gate if you like, but I prefer this little stunt with the garden wall.

'No news on great granddad's cup yet,' I say.

'Oh,' she chews on her gums, teeth already out and in the glass beside her.

Great-grandfather Wild on my mother's side was a seafaring man with the East India Company, which seems to me a magnificent thing to have been. Granny doesn't know much about him but she has passed on to me a couple of his things – a dress sword and silver cup awarded to him, together with a beautiful thank-you letter in copperplate, for a lifetime of service. Heinously, I am now trying to sell the silver cup. I'm still in debt at the bank, it's taking a long time to pay off and I need money for Falmouth. I'm starting afresh at Falmouth. In fact this idea of selling off a family heirloom to quickly raise some funds has been on my mind for a while, and was first mooted with De Gruyter the day he visited Colham in the winter. Lise said he would help, that he was good at this kind of thing and would get me a good price. I took the plunge, got the cup out and polished it up with Duraglit – a splendid item, a ceremonial chalice, all rococo chasing and scrolls, with a dolphin on the lid, gilt-lined inside. But I had no attachment to it. I found it gross. I told Granny about my imminent crime and she only said 'If it helps …', and Mum and Frank didn't object either. So, before starting at Debenhams, I packed up just about the only piece of family silver and went up to De Gruyter's house in West London to flog it. We went round the local antique shops together. He did the talking. Everyone seemed interested – though they didn't like to know that we'd tried elsewhere – and offered around thirty pounds for it. I was happy with that, but De Gruyter had seen the glint in their eyes and said I should try Sotheby's. They accepted the cup with alacrity and said they would let me know.

I keep Granny updated. Though she would probably have preferred me to keep it, she's impressed by the name of the auction house. She has always been interested in trading antiques, Granny. A sale of early Victorian silver will eventually take place in the autumn and my great grandfather's cup will sell for a hundred and eighty pounds. Thank you, Granny and De Gruyter. But of course the money won't arrive for about another year and doesn't help present cash flow problems.

A few days after Granny's escapade with the police, I'm writing: *Life has hit rock bottom. What am I doing? Nothing that has any meaning. I wander emptily around at work all day ... The evenings are free but what to do with them? I sit in my room, smoke, daydream about the past, and less often the future. I see no future – no romance. Feel so oppressed by home. Know no one. Pete, the lodger next door, I could go and see – perhaps I will. I met him by chance on a walk ten days ago and have been avoiding the issue. Must stick out work for another week and a half. Can't move until I've got some money. Then all hopes are pinned on Falmouth, a new home, new people, fresh purpose.*

I go down to Falmouth in August, several weeks early. The bus into Taunton, the pleasant, meandering train journey. For the third time this year I get out on the friendly platform of the Dell and walk into town. It's the height of the holiday season now and the place is packed, traffic nosing through the people, everywhere the reek of fried food, the squawking din of gulls. Just up the hill from the heaving harbour and not far from the college, straightaway, serendipitously, I see a ROOM TO LET sign in the window of a tall slate-clad town house. A spindly, aproned, mischievous woman shows me the large ground floor room at the back, just a lean-to extension that smells strongly of damp, but there's a skylight and a small rampant garden. This will do fine. 11 Swanpool Street will be my address for the next two years. My new landlady Mrs Birch shows me her walled garden stuffed with southern and semi-tropical plants: an echium fifteen-foot tall, bottle brushes, rampant fuchsias, succulents, ferns, and two eucalyptus trees 'which grow and grow', she ho-hos. Several dachshunds run yapping round my feet.

I walk around the seaside town, which is quite large, and away from the long winding main street, quieter. It strings itself along one side of the River Fal with many hundreds of small craft of all descriptions swinging and bobbing at anchor; there's a small, enticing ferry across to the village of Flushing on the other side. And Jacob's Ladder, an extraordinarily precipitous flight of 111 stone steps to the upper town, made by a local builder to link the lower and upper town so he could get to his properties more easily.

That first night I go out to a wine bar by the harbour front and end up in a corner alone. Back in the sanctuary of my room, I blab in a notebook:

I see myself through other people in this intensely self-critical way. Seem to be conscious of myself every moment of the day. In three weeks time I start at the art school and I'm scared. I'm trapped pencil in hand, having to create something. These last few days I've been forcing myself to draw. I feel that I can do nothing else but at the same time can't even do this.

I wish my pen could flow so smoothly the words would appear as quickly as the thoughts – it nearly does every now and then. Then I could get it all down in one stream and look back at it. You have to be so careful or the words don't come out truthfully. I'm indulging myself now, allowing everything to come to the surface. I spend the day fighting it, keeping it down, in a continuous effort to keep afloat. 'Till human voices wake us and we drown.' I wish something would happen to me out of my control, an accident of some kind, so I would have to go into hospital ...

The next two pages are glued together so thoroughly I can't unstick them, and no doubt go on in similar vein. I'm twenty-one, adult, everything going for me, yet under this weight. I can see no reason for it, or everything is a reason. I return to

Wellington after only a couple of days and find things aren't any better there. Frank persuades me to go to the doctor, who gives me Valium and probably something else. Our Dr Richardson was quite a pill-pusher in those liberal days. His pen was poised over the pad when you went in; he'd prescribe aspirin and paracetemol *because* they were free. I take the Valium and feel calm again. He told me to stop thinking, fighting and bashing myself. That seems to be what's happening. I note, 'Five days under sedation from Dr R. Got up feeling better today and wanted to go to Reading to start house decorating.'

For a little problem has arisen. My father has invited Clare and me (not Catherine for some reason) to his new house in Reading to decorate it. This is in part a substitute for our lost summer holiday at Colham. A paid holiday with Dad is most attractive – any holiday with him would be good; a bit of patient caustic soda stripping of a piece of pine would surely work well with the Valium. But I'm in a quandary. I can't go to like this. My father mustn't see me in this drugged state. I must always go to his place well and happy. This fresh collapse … it's like one of my mother's, for God's sake. It's mental. (Ah, how like *his* mother this sounds.) I fret over it in my diary: *We are meant to be going today …* Does Clare go first and I follow when I'm 'more settled'? Does she delay for me? We do go in the end, because this is when we paint Dad's famous 'brown hall', a glossy saddle-brown that remains to this day. All the doors, staircase, skirting, the old embossed 'pub' wallpaper up to dado rail, a job seems to go on forever, an infinity of fumy sticky oil paint. Then Dad tops it off with spotlights, creating a marvellous chiarascuro effect with the lights reflecting off the high gloss. It becomes his 'Caravaggio' hall and all the more magical for that.

Part Two: Falmouth

12. Try again

My room in Swanpool Street is five minutes from the Art School. On a Monday morning in late September I walk up to Woodside and sign in. The admin buildings are at the top of the hill, the studios below them among sub-tropical gardens. I'm feeling better now. The drugs have worked or the mood has passed. I'm off them anyway. It's good to be in a seaside town, the harbour a minute away down the hill, the beaches a short walk into the afternoon sun and sunset; the amazing sight of oil tankers creeping into the bay to anchor their huge hulks in the docks, the never-ending cacophony of gulls on rooftops, and still bustling crowds anywhere near the water. I've started an oil painting in my room and it's going okay. I'm going to paint in oils here in Falmouth.

First-years assemble in the painting studios with tutors Francis Hewlett and Dick Platt and we launch into a discussion of what art's all about. I feel I know where much of this is going. Actually we're talking about a branch of painting, the post-war Euston Road School. Hewlett is a Euston Road painter, Coldstream-taught like Mum and Dad. He's an 'objective' painter: his aim to be truthful to the image in front of him. He thinks it would be a good idea if all those interested in painting did this for a while: work with him, learn how to paint objectively, then go off and do what you like. Nature, says Hewlett, is infinitely interesting, surprising and inspiring. Just look at it. The more you look, the more you'll see. You can't go wrong by taking a hard look at what's in front of you and painting that.

'You've got these beautiful gardens, the harbour and boats, all the landscapes of Cornwall, and there'll be a model coming in to pose most weeks,' he says.

This back-to-basics, work-from-nature approach is more or

less what he told me at my interview. ('There's much of interest in your portfolio but put it aside for a year. Paint objectively.') After the vagueness and anything goes of Reading, I'm happy to go along with it – I want to be told what to do. Anyway I *have* come here to paint from nature. I'm continuing from where I left off in the spring in the Colham valley. But others say, 'Life drawing?'

'Painting from the model in a white studio?'

'Painting, period!'

Painting from life on canvas on old-fashioned easels in the studio isn't what people do now, according to half the people in the room. This suddenly feels like Reading in reverse. Now it's the tutors wanting us to learn to paint the old way, while the new ideas pour in from the students. What about photography and film? What about installations? Performance? Dance? How about some *ideas*? All those ideas that were around when I was at Reading are still around, and bigger, stronger now.

'Well, I teach painting from life,' says Hewlett. 'And that's what some of us are here to do. You might think of the *optimism* of the Impressionists when you're down here in Cornwall painting *plein air*.'

We separate into painters and sculptors; painters staying put, sculptors going up to their own studios. The ones who don't want to be in either group veer towards sculpture. Sculpture is less confining. Later on they will subdivide into photographers, film-makers, printmakers, potters, textilers, 'conceptualists', and one writer.

I get a drawing board and stock of paper, pencils and charcoal from the college shop. I replenish my oil paints. Materials are very cheap – a wodge of A1 cartridge paper costs next to nothing. John the technician, a sailor from Dartmouth, advises buying cotton duck canvas off the roll for economy, and making our own stretchers; the wood in the carpentry workshop is free for that purpose. I put the materials in the studio by my allotted easel. There will be a life model coming in later in the week or next week and I'll give it a go. But what now? I don't feel inclined to work in the sterile white studio any more than I did at Reading. Nor do I have to. I ask Dick about working at home in my room, where I already have something on the go.

'That's f-fine. Bring it in to show us,' he stammers. Dick is kind and helpful, always, though some will call him soft.

The painting is a reflection of my room in a mirror. I've propped the mirror on the table, giving a reflection of most of the room, angled so I'm not in it. I like the idea of this condensed image of my room. I also quickly discover, usefully, how the elements of the picture are simplified by being in two dimensions. In the mirror image everything is already on a flat plane and so much easier to transfer to the canvas. I use the colours that appear to me to be right, which I realise later are almost entirely in the blue/orange contrast. In fact I find the painting very easy, it has a flow of its own.

After a couple of days I take it in to show them. Dick admires the colour. 'I love that t-turquoise with the brown and orange!'

Turquoise? I don't let on. I accept the praise. Pure luck, of course. By mixing blue into the 'shadow' I've come up with this startling blue-green. The painting comes home and I do some more work on it – and ruin it, apparently. But I don't think that. I think the widening out and crisping of the edges, the flattening of table surface and lightening the colours, are improvements. I spend some time on the bevelling of the mirror, which has an interesting prismatic effect as the sun moves round the room. But I've lost the flash of turquoise, that rather magical colour effect, Dick says, disappointed next time he sees it. I have lost the colour I can't actually see. This is all rather difficult – I can't set out to create these chance colour effects, can I? I *am* painting objectively, aren't I?

Second-year painter Charlotte has an upstairs room at Swanpool Street. She's the only other lodger at the moment. Wavy brown hair, nice brown eyes, she spends a lot of time painting in her room too. Alone is not the same as lonely, we agree, meeting every now and then in the kitchen. We like to work on our own, we're allies in shunning the studios. We can do better, work all the hours we like, all night if we want. She's painting her denim jacket hung on a hook on the back of her door. Unprepossessing subject, yet a fascinating painting. The frayed blue denim, the brass studs and buttons, the gleam of the gloss paint on the door itself, she has made so real. She works by electric light for constancy and has caught that lurid quality of light too. The painting is so straight and unadorned, concentrated – all very truthful somehow. I admire the small intense canvas on her easel in the centre of the room.

'Get yourself an easel,' she advises. 'They don't mind.'

So I bring back my easel from the studios. From now on I will be tripping over its three splayed legs day and night.

One night Charlotte and I go for a walk to the town beach. A warm wind laden with the smells of drying seaweed is blowing off the sea, the waves breaking white on the low-tide rocks. We sit on the shingle at the back beach and kiss. She doesn't want to go any further. Not now. She doesn't have anyone at the moment but doesn't want anyone. She's sorry – it isn't me. Of course it *is* me, but still, as we walk back to our rooms, the air clears between us. And thus it remains. We settle into easy friendship, painters side by side. I do notice though, as you do, that she's a long time without a relationship, and when at last it happens, it's serious and lasting, and with the Art History lecturer.

On the first turn of the stairs hangs a remarkable painting by an ex-student, John Magoldrick. Mrs Birch acquired it instead of rent. 'Oh, the boy went off somewhere and left this behind.

He had some troubles, poor boy,' she indicates with a finger on her temple. Yes, she agrees, it is rather good, she's glad she didn't throw it out. Just a corner of white screen, paint table, window, the lawn outside. The real subject is light. No lines at all, just thick swirling paint, bright and light. He's made so much out of his dull old studio space. He's filled it with joy somehow. I see this light-filled vision every time I go upstairs to the bathoom.

In the studios there's a painter called Kate. She seems to be a landscape painter. That's to say her first painting in the studio is a landscape (well, seascape). She's gamine like Charlotte, more so – you could say Audrey Hepburn with a bit of Artful Dodger – an intense and serious girl from North London with a lisp. I find she's easy to talk to, we click. And I see immediately how well she can paint. This seascape of hers already seems to be head and shoulders above anyone else's in the year. It's of Gyllyngvase beach at low tide, rocks draped with heaps of stinking bladder wrack, sea and sky dark; the sombre tones laid on flat, strong, horizontal. She works thickly with a palette knife and will boldly scrape the whole lot off next morning, build it up again. There's no preciousness about her work. She's after Hewlett's truth to the landscape, just as Charlotte is with her still life of the denim jacket.

Simon is an approachable guy. Also from London, his father an architect with the GLC. Coincidentally, Simon went to Leighton Park School in Reading, just by the university campus. He's short, wiry black-haired, olive-skinned, a rather quiet figure in the background. But after a drink he explodes into life, he suddenly becomes the extrovert, does handstands and cartwheels on the pavement outside the pub like some acrobat, man of the circus. If the subject of my art is still life, then Simon's is the human figure. He's waiting for life-drawing to start, and when it does he will stick with it. All his work will be about drawing and painting the model. He will study anatomy, the movement of the body. When the model has gone home, I'll find him at work on a drab-coloured painting – the colours of the screens, the splattered floorboards, the model's couch or chair, always seemed so drab and dirty to me – with sketches from the model pinned up, a fan of brushes and palette in his hand, squinting at his canvas. Simon puts in long hours and is reliably there to talk to when I've spent too long alone in my room. He also has one of the few college rooms, handily nearby, and I go back with him to listen to David Bowie and The Spiders from Mars.

Thom from Austria, tall and black-bearded, has shrugged off all this 'drawing from life' from the start. He is more interested in photographing people's reactions to a fifty-pence piece he has glued to the pavement in the busy part of town. He's an ideas man, a conceptualist. Thom's lines of thought are closer to Edward de Bono's – and thus very enviable. Lateral Thinking is meat and drink for his original mind. As I've said, I struggled with the balancing of knives on milk bottles, the subtlety and nuance of the solution. Edward de Bono and Thom's thoughts seem to pick up just where mine stop. I would like to make that jump, get my mind to bend and stretch like that.

Pasters, the bishop's son, is the comedian of our year. To my mind an actor, to his a musician, the drummer in a band he's starting up. Pasters plays the fool. With me he plays the Man with the Stiff Upper Lip, greeting me with a loud 'Froy, how *is it*, you fruit bat?' He himself hasn't actually started on any work yet, has a bit of trouble getting *down* to art …

Just as garrulous is bearded, passionate Joseph from Belfast. 'Dunno about you lot of *fine* artists here, but I'm from the Bogside, *amn't I*,' he challenges in his Derry brogue, 'and now I'm living on *thee* bloody Cornish Riviera. And *what* am I going to do about home?' He talks about Northern Ireland, the violence, the war situation since Bloody Sunday. He juxtaposes this place of fancy tropical gardens and whatnot. So why did he come here? I think he'll have trouble reconciling three years 'painting from the model' with the turmoil in Bogside.

I go to life drawing. Kate goes. Simon's there. Joseph is doing some rough charcoal drawings. Most of us have a go, though not Thom. The model Suzanne has long ginger hair to her waist and sharp teeth. She's completely at ease with her neat body – of course she is, stripping off and being scrutinized day in day out. And here we all are, standing around her, clothed, staring at her.

We do quick poses. A minute or two to sketch the whole figure. No time to get precious or fussy about the work, already on to the next one, a fresh sheet of paper clipped to the board, working large and free. She's standing, crouching, bending, stretching with hands clasped above her head. I work in charcoal like Joseph, smear the paper with my fingers, loose and ill-defined, tones rather than lines. The human body is very difficult to draw.

Then it's slowed right down. We have all morning, several mornings, with one pose. Hewlett is here and guiding us through objective drawing: plot the various points of the figure on the paper, measure by holding the pencil out at arm's length and, squinting, transfer the distances to the paper. If it helps, look through a grid to get the measurements like the old masters. In any case, keep your head still to maintain the same viewpoint. And try not to use an eraser. Draw 'honestly', leave all the marks you make on the paper. They are part of the integrity of the drawing.

Back at Swanpool Street I have another go at being objective, for discipline. I make a careful pencil drawing of my room with ruled lines of perspective, with all the little pointers and marks left in. I squint and plot, apply the same rigour of position and viewpoint to the space of my room: the bed, cabinet, sloping ceiling, window. At least I find this inanimate subject matter easier to manage than the live flesh of the model. But I never make a painting of it. It isn't important to me. It seems contrived and uninvolving. Maybe I'm just undisciplined. I continue to work with a sharp pencil for a while.

13. Swanpool Street interior

Autumn is coming on and my 'garden' room gets cold. The only source of heating is a smelly paraffin stove, which I keep going all day with gallons of paraffin from the hardware shop – the jerrycan and funnel sit in the corner and no doubt constitute a serious fire hazard. There is an ancient, unusable cast iron range built into the wall in my room. With its rust and detailed ironwork, it will later become the subject of a painting. But my second Swanpool Street interior is of the curtained windows looking out on the garden. I complete one window with curtains either side, then decide to make it a double canvas, a diptych, with both windows linked by the curtains. Thinking of Charlotte's truthful denim jacket, I spend a lot of time on the sheeny pattern and texture of those curtains – like an old master, like Velasquez (let's say something like a small Velasquez plate in an art book). I love painting the light on the satiny blue and cream curtains, the shadows blue and brown. I have some problems with the plants in the garden, the greens going heavy on me. How I long to produce a clear living green, a green that's true to nature. I put in Mrs Birch, so often to be found out there bending over her plants, thin and hawkish, silver-haired. I fancifully give her a black jersey and a string of pearls.

Swanpool Street Interior 2 does less well under the Platt scrutiny. He thinks the colour isn't as good – not so lucky this time, I think. But he's happy for me to continue painting in this vein in my room. He seems to hold out great hopes for me.

This painting has survived. Mum claimed it after I left Falmouth and put it up on her bedroom wall, where it remains, though she has long gone.

It's surprising how little Charlotte and I meet in the kitchen.

Maybe she's trying to discourage any further advances from me. Or perhaps we just don't coincide – I think she eats like a bird. Maybe she's avoiding the new lodger, Dave. I see plenty of Dave, a lugubrious Yorkshireman who has come down to Falmouth to do the special boat-building course at the Tech. Dave hangs around the kitchen hoping to talk to people; he's lurking there when I go to make a quick cup of coffee. He takes me up to the attic to see his boat plans, which I don't find very interesting, not at this time – they are nothing to do with Art. Later, when I'm living on a Pacific island, boat dependent, the world of yachts will have very much more relevance.

I have Elizabeth David's *French Provincial Cooking*, which my father uses, and Granny Helen uses, and I am keen to follow. I'm still very much a learner. Dad taught me how to make a spag bol, that bastion of male cooking, years ago. Anna in Bedford showed me how to improvise on that, make your bol sauce the basis for any number of dishes. I've made myself a Frank-style egg and bacon supper often enough. Frank says he could eat egg and bacon every night, and is liable to quote Wittgenstein in this respect: 'I'll eat anything as long as it's the same.' But I'd like my supper to be different every night. I like the business of cooking and infinite variation. I'm starting to refine it, see the art in it.

Eggs are cheap and omelettes have begun to feature in my diet. I follow David's instructions: Don't beat the eggs to death but *stir* them with two forks; lightness is everything in omelettes. I learn the business of tilting the pan back and forth, gathering and folding the mixture as it cooks and sets. At home Frank often cooks omelettes. Besides being simple and cheap, they are Mum's favourite. When he married Mum she said she'd be happy with an omelette with a green salad and glass of red wine every night, he never tires of telling us.

And fish. I've discovered you can get a mackerel off the fishing boats for as little as five pence. They are absolutely fresh and delicious. But first I've had to overcome them. Not the messy gutting and cleaning, which I've never minded, but my apparent allergy to some kinds. As a child I was unable to tolerate any of the oily fish – sprats, pilchards, herrings, mackerel – and sicked them up without fail. I grew to fear them, couldn't stand the smell of them frying in the house. Since leaving home I've continued to avoid 'fishy fish'. You don't want to spend good money and then throw it up. So I grill my first, straight-off-the-boat, quay-fresh, five pence mackerel with some trepidation; eat it gingerly with plenty of bread, and it stays down. Probably all to do with the freshness of the fish but I'm actually overjoyed my childhood affliction is going. During my three years in Cornwall I will build a tolerance, an understanding, with mackerel and then sardines (herrings stay iffy the longest). Necessity is the mother of many things.

There is only one fixture in the week, the History of Art/Complementary Studies lecture. Tim Holiday's art history is orthodox European from the Impressionists onwards. Lionel Miskin's is a meander through the world's art in search of Jungian Universals and Archetypes, comparative art, the art of symbols. He's interested in everything, his talks are passionate, all-encompassing. They lean towards the sexual.

'Look at this Peruvian pot phallus. Extraordinary! These New Guinea penis sheathes the chaps still wear, apparently. Fascinating!'

He patrols the room, lanky, preoccupied, faces us with his frown and long bushy moustache, spreads his thin arms wide, runs back to the projector and shows us slides of Polynesian, Eskimo and Tibetan art. Juxtaposes a Lascaux cave painting with a Picasso bull. Up pops a Nigerian bronze head.

'Now look at these Earth Mothers!' He clicks on to a little stone fertility goddess from Neolithic Germany, which he puts beside a massive Henry Moore sculpture, which in turn is like a flint nodule the artist picked up in St Margaret's Bay, Dover.

'Anyone know the notion Gaia?'

It's the first time I've heard the word Gaia, the name coined, revived, by the writer William Golding just a few years ago (1969), and I feel a great affinity with it. I love the idea of the earth as a self-regulating living entity, love the idea of an earth mother – my own mother seems very far from this. Earth mothers, I think, aren't constantly needy and demanding and misbehaving, they are the providers, the regulators. I will dabble with religions in Cornwall, call myself a Pantheist for a while, by which I really mean I want my god to be all of nature. Gaia can do that for me.

In the attic of Woodside, I find the Photography Department and the bushy-bearded, twinkly-eyed bundle of energy that is Wilk. I want to photograph some oystercatchers on the beach and Wilk hands me a 35 mm camera with a telephoto lens and a tripod. He shows me how to use a through-the-lens camera, gives me a black and white film, a fairly fast one, 400ASA, for the job, which will gain on the light but lose on the fineness of detail. 'No need to stint on film,' he says. 'You're here to take pictures, so take plenty. No one's counting here.' I can use up a whole roll of film on oystercatchers on a winter beach if I want. I'm shown how to reuse a film cassette: unroll a length from the 100-metre roll and feed it into a cassette spool, a tricky and delicate operation, carried out 'blind' in a black bag. Then you have a fresh film for next to nothing. It's all very generous and unprecious.

I stalk my oystercatchers out on the low tide rocks, slippery with bladder wrack and kelp. Snap the birds from too far away, get closer, snap them again, until at some signal they simultaneously take flight. There are turnstones among them, and purple sandpipers – a new species for me. Fulmars glide past on their stiff wings, even here on the town beach and headland. Fulmars are interesting, on the increase, recolonising the whole of Britain now. I'm keen on birds again.

I bring back my film and Wilk teaches me about the darkroom. When the exposed film comes out of the camera the room must be pitch black, no chinks of light anywhere, but for the rest of the time the red light can be on – the special red bulb – and by then your eyes are accustomed and there is enough light to see. We develop the film and peg up the sticky negative strips to dry. Next day we print a contact sheet, all the pictures on one sheet like thumbnails, and select which ones to enlarge. He thinks I have a couple of good shots of the flying oystercatchers. In the eerie glow of the darkroom it is immensely satisfying to see the magical process of a picture appearing before my eyes in the bath of developer. I print experimentally on different grades of paper, hard and soft, contrasty and grainy, for various effects.

Longing for my own SLR camera, my grant cheque freshly arrived, I blow a hole in it by buying a secondhand Yashica from the camera shop in town. A giddying experience – this is so much money – but, as we say now, I had to have it. I make my purchase, emerge from the shop triumphant. This 'spending to the hilt', though reined in, has never fully left me. It's a recklessness my mother has, and she says she got it from her father. The Yashica will serve me well for many years – it pays for itself – until I see that Pentax in a duty-free shop in Panama City. Then I stretch to a Nikon, an old manual one, but what a fine lens. Then it all goes digital …

I continue to borrow all the telephoto lenses I want from Wilk, as well as specialist items such as lens filters and a cable release. I spend a lot of time in Wilk's photography department among the strong formaldehyde smells of developer and fixative. Thom is often up there. He's printing a whole series of people trying to get his glued down 50p off the pavement. One day I'm grumbling to him about being overworked doing two degrees – my Open University Ecology assignments are now arriving thick and fast in the post.

'Pushing yourself to the limit never hurt anyone,' says Wilk sharply.

But I'm going off the idea. Why am I doubling up like this? The basic science, before we even reach any ecology, has become a burden. It clashes with painting all the time. With painting, I've realised, I like to spend *all* my time, immerse myself. There just isn't the time for the science. Wilk helps keep me going with the OU for a while longer but I will soon give it up. Ditch the ecology. Concentrate energy. Be an artist, I tell myself.

Kate has stopped work on her beach painting. It remains unchanged on her easel for days. I tell her how much I admire it, the thick creamy oil paint, the rich dark colour, the confidence in laying it on the canvas.

'Like a de Staël,' I say.

'I'm finished with painting,' she says. 'Giving it up. Makes me sick.'

An astonishing statement. After just one painting here, and a really good one. In her dogged lisping voice, she explains that she was out on Pendennis Point and actually sick thinking about paint. 'The smell of it, the feel of it!' She's certain she can't go on with it.

And she does give it up. By the end of the term, Kate has stopped painting and taken up writing. She works with writer-in-residence Paddy Kitchen and then with the poet Peter Redgrove when he gets back from the States. She sticks with Redgrove and after three years will present for her degree show just several large foolscap books filled with dense tiny writing – automatic writing, dream writing, fantasy writing, a non-stop outpouring of writing. She'll get a First for it and apply for the now-famous 'original' creative writing course at the University of East Anglia.

It's the Christmas party, the art school dance. For this I make myself a pair of owlish glasses out of card, colour them a livid green, and tape them to my own glasses – a mask and disguise. I'm going as a camp Mr Hockney. Up in Simon's room, the great exhibitionist David Bowie is thumping out his *Diamond Dogs*. I borrow some make-up, someone helps me with mascara; I moue my lips and put the outrageous glasses back on. It's all very earnest. The done thing for blokes here is to indulge in a little risqué dressing up in these androgynous times. I remember my father saying how he hated the androgynous Bowie, but that was what I liked about him! At future parties I'll borrow a dress and go in full drag, an early version of the artist Grayson Perry in his frocks, perhaps. We go to the disco dance in the canteen and common room. Simon is a jester, the character he will adopt as his alter ego at Falmouth. While he springs and clowns his way around the dance floor, I drink myself silly, then prance like a madman. I don't get off with anyone. If the object was to let my hair down that's fine, but if it was to find a girl, it might not have been so helpful to dress up as a semi-tranny Hockney.

My father comes down to Cornwall for Christmas – Colham is still let. Dad, Catherine H and Francesca, and my sisters Clare and Catherine. With Charlotte's help I've found a holiday cottage on the Lizard Peninsula.

The cottage, in the village of Ruan Minor above Cadgwith, is damp and mildewy, with musty sofas, but with the weather so mild, we can spend the days outside. I draw the rough stone church with its detached stubby tower, the churchyard of wind-bent trees. The tiny church down in Cadgwith Cove is blue-painted tin, like a shed with a cross perched on top.

Cornwall is full of such vernacular architecture. My sketch of St. Ruan's has survived the vicissitudes of forty years; I like its easy, unselfconscious scribble.

On New Year's Day there's an expedition to Sennen Cove at Land's End, where my father comes into his own. He gets everything shipshape, into packs and baskets, all we might need. We climb down to a great beach of white sand. There, he deploys us to collect wood and mussels; the small blue-black mussels cover the rocks in their thousands. Dad can make something special out of such a simple thing as collecting a few shellfish and boiling them up in seawater on a driftwood fire. We all join in, being kids again. I light the fire with as few matches as possible, as though I'll get a prize for it. We prepare thick slices of bread and butter and wait for the tiny, beardy, delicious mussels.

Then we call in at Terry Frost's house in Newlyn for tea. I find my father knows Terry well. Their careers have tracked each other since the fifties: consecutive Gregory Fellows in Leeds (Dad first), both teachers at Reading (Terry first). I remember Terry's vivid slide show at Reading. Though an abstract painter, he said all his inspiration came from nature: suns, moons, boats, reflections. Now I can see how his 'colours and curves' might derive from boats rocking and jostling in a Cornish harbour, colourful bodies in a crowded winding street. But these are abstractions he has reached after years: I'm a figurative painter, I'm sticking to what I see. But then again my drawing of the church contains a whole lot of abstract scribbles that stand for the bare branches in the wind.

Frost has an ebullience, a tremendous *joie de vivre*, which makes us Froys seem rather small and timid. He has a fascinating tale to tell about his prisoner-of-war experience: 'Prison camp was my university … I got tremendous spiritual experience, a more aware and heightened perception during starvation, and I honestly think that awakening has never left me.' He was captured in Crete in 1941, incarcerated in several camps, and ended up in Stalag 383 in Bavaria with the artist Adrian Heath, who taught him how to paint. They remained there for the rest of the war, not devising ways of escape but ways of painting. They made brushes out of horsehair, canvases from pillows, mixed what pigments they could get with the oil from sardine cans. Here, surely, are heroes as worthy as the Great Escapers I was brought up on; most people in prison camps just got on with the business of surviving, struggling to marginally improve their lives and those of their fellow prisoners. Meanwhile, Kurt Schwitters, interned as an alien on the Isle of Man, was also working with ever-increasing ingenuity in his camp, tearing up lino floors to work on, making sculpture from porridge. After the war Frost decided to be a painter, and with Heath's help got an ex-serviceman's grant to go to art school. He devoted the rest of his life to art.

'Kazwasti!' he cried, whatever that meant.

I also note now how Terry was freed in April 1945 and married that same August, a union which would last until his death in 2002 and bring six children. There are six children in our family too, but from four marriages.

I enjoyed the brilliance and ebullience of our visit to Terry Frost's house and studio overlooking Newlyn Harbour, but it's also true to say I resisted going to tea with my father's artist friends, with its whiff of nepotism. I'd had enough of that at Reading. I was still trying to get away from my artist family.

14. Rhapsodic

They have all gone back. Dad and co. to their new house in Reading, Clare to her second term at the Slade, Catherine to her second term at Taunton Tech. I can still feel homesick at twenty-one. I take my binoculars and head out to the cliffs of my new Cornish home. It's windy but not cold. Cornwall gets this wonderful warm wind without rain, or preceding rain, the warmth swept up from the Azores. A left turn at the beaches goes up to Henry VIII's Pendennis Castle – where Kate came to her momentous decision to give up painting. A right turn leads west to the headland of Pennance Point. It's wilder here, thrilling to be high above the churning sea. As a very young child I loved to run out of the house to the common, a 'windy boyser'. I can do the same now, run and spread my arms wide, buffeted by the warm damp wind. The trees on the cliff grow twisted and bent-backed. Gulls and stiff-winged fulmars hang in the wind at cliff-top level. I lie on my stomach in the wiry grass to steady the binoculars and search among the rocks for the black redstarts that live along here. It will take several visits to find them but six months later my diary joyfully confirms: 9 *November. Black Redstart! Male. On the low cliffs, one clear view only. Black throat, dark back with white wing patches, rusty flicking tail.*

I take my drawing board out to the point, sketch its tree-covered hulk against the westering light. I like to draw trees in winter, their transparency against the dark line of the land, their intricate tangle of branches.

If anything it seems to be damper inside buildings than outside. In my room the January damp gets everywhere. Clothes, bedding, books, paper, all smell of mould and must. I keep the smelly paraffin stove burning. It mingles with oil paint, linseed, white spirit in the room. I sit on the warm stove, smoking, adding to the cocktail of fumes, and contemplate my drawing of Pennance Point.

Through the steamed up window, Mrs Birch is out in her garden. With no frost, or almost no frost, gardening can go on year round here. She's planting two more eucalyptus seedlings, making four in this small space. Under her loving green fingers they will soon be giants. The neighbours will be round, she sighs and giggles – she can't stop planting things. She potters around her pots and nursery of plants outside my room all day. Knocks on the door and reads me a letter from her hippy son Robin in Ireland, who is apparently living the life of Riley in a gypsy caravan out on the west coast. She tells me about her cousin John Seymour, who is writing a book on 'living off the land' that might interest me. It does and I read *Self -Sufficiency*, a forerunner of this now common genre: 'Are you one of the growing army of people in the cities and in the country who deplore the modern methods of food production and would like to do something about it for themselves?' I also read E.F. Schumacher's *Small is Beautiful*. Now here's something to believe in. Everything Schumacher says in his book seems so absolutely clear and obvious to me. Of course things should be done on a small, local, intimate scale. Of course economics should be 'as if people mattered'. To try and live our lives 'beautifully, on a small scale' is why so many of us have come down to Cornwall.

Mrs Birch's oddjob man David arrives to discuss glassing over the area outside my door so that she can grow yet more tender plants. David can turn his hand to anything. Together, outside my door, they design a glass and wood structure that will withstand the gales. He's an odd-looking man with no eyelashes. I feel his lizard eyes on me, appraising me; I meet his gaze, offer no response. I pointedly ignore these 'gay' winks; I do not allow him to linger chatting on the threshold of my room and firmly close the door. He goes off to get building materials for the job and returns with some enormous sheets of glass, which he cuts into triangles and rhomboid shapes to fit the space. 'Not a right angle to be found at Mrs B's!' he quips. 'But you can always cut to fit, John.' David is often around, fixing things in the house and garden and he ceases to be a threat. I have no idea that I will become something of an odd-jobber like him.

I paint to classical music. Pop is for evenings and going out. I have my little cassette recorder, some homemade cassette tapes of my own, and many more from Frank. Frank is now recording copiously from the radio. He has made me a Segovia tape I treasure. Segovia, still playing at the age of 81, is the greatest classical guitarist of all, Frank informs me, adding an anecdote – he has one for every composer, conductor and soloist: 'Segovia said he only had three wives and three guitars in his life but he flirted with others.' Although our tastes will end up quite different – his cerebral, mine romantic, perhaps – Frank has a great influence on my growing musical discrimination. He loves the big sopranos, his 'canary birds', Maria Callas and Joan Sutherland, whom at the time I just find shrieky. He has his opera divas on tape and it can be alarming at home when some famous 'mad scene' comes from his room, while the real thing, more or less, is going on with Mum downstairs.

I have a recording of the *Goldberg Variations* played by Wanda Landowska, which Frank also admires. He told me the story of the heavy, metal harpsichord Landowska had had specially made. Built like a piano with strings an octave below normal pitch, it had gone right out of fashion. When the great cellist Pablo Casals criticised her heavy-handed playing of this instrument, she retorted 'You play Bach your way, and I'll play him his way.' Of course I'm far less discerning – for a start I have nothing to compare it with. To me it's just louder and stronger than other harpsichords. I don't remember Glenn Gould's performances being available then or Frank would surely have suggested them.

He points me towards Beethoven's late quartets, which go right over my head; I'm happy enough just to get to grips with the nine symphonies. When I discover Schubert, he gives me acclaimed recordings of *Death and the Maiden* and the *Trout*; Schubert has remained exquisite. Dear Frank, his letters from home, so often centred round my mother and her current crimes and misdemeanours, often include snippets, like little pleas for sanity, from his great knowledge of music.

My classical guitar lives in the corner of the room – another smell: sweet cedar every time I open its red felt-lined case. I practise earnestly, keep on with the classical pieces I've taken up with Catherine H at Colham. I become enamoured of Llobet's exquisite *El Testamen de N'Amelia* and play it with exaggerated vibrato. I spend a great number of hours on something that I will abandon, as with so many things.

Frank gives me T.S. Eliot's *Collected Poems* 1909-1962 for my birthday. He gives a book each birthday of my Falmouth years – seminal books for me: *The Popular Handbook of British Birds*, Philip Larkin's *High Windows*. I already know *Prufrock* from Dad's recital at Colham, now I learn the poem by heart. I love *Ash-Wednesday* and the *Four Quartets*. I love *Rhapsody on a Windy Night*, which to me suggests a euphoric walk along the cliffs to Pennance Point as much as a stagger home from the pub under yellow streetlights.

I love *High Windows* too, find these poems completely accessible. For me Philip Larkin has always been entwined with Frank. Their shared bluntness, rude humour, atheism. Larkin, the non-believer in his cycle clips, tours English parish churches for their architecture like Frank; they both enter damp empty places of worship, hollow steps on cold stone, realistically – it's a potent image. This pottering around local churches has of course been much practised by others such as John Betjeman, and is the *sine qua non* of the non-religious, church-visiting Nikolaus Pevsner – two more of my stepfather's heroes.

Robert Pirsig's book *Zen and the Art of Motorcycle Maintenance*, another life-changer on my shelves, is actually Frank's brother Bert's recommendation. Bert, a microbiologist at Cambridge, was doing a doctorate in Honolulu. He became interested in Zen, and friends with Zen Master Katsuki Sekida, while he was there and wrote the introductions to two of Sekida's books. Frank later pointed out that these books had never been out of print. If you're going to write, he said, do something that lasts, like a textbook. But then he was a school teacher all his working life. I note now that Pirsig's book was initially rejected by 121 publishers, a record for a best-seller, according to the *Guinness Book of Records*. At Falmouth, its theme of being at one with machines, knowing how they work, how to dismantle and reassemble them, while respecting them, their *nature*, I try to live by. When I get a motorbike (of sorts) in my third year, I maintain it. At last I learn the ins and outs of a simple engine. I become more or less at one with my machine. Of course this is all pre-microchip. Since machines became electronic there has been no chance of my understanding them.

I treasure my *Handbook* of British Birds, my 'Witherby', from Frank, a large hardback volume. I start a life checklist of birds in its endpapers. It still possesses a fine, musty Swanpool Street smell.

There are plenty of birds to see locally around Falmouth, the headlands and beaches, the many muddy tidal creeks. For fresh ticks I need go no further than Swanpool Beach and its productive lagoon. One Sunday morning of bright sun and north wind, I chance on a group of birders with their telescopes and gear. We see: a rare Iceland gull, a rare Mediterranean gull, sandwich terns, a great northern diver, three Slavonian grebes, one with its handsome summer orange plume. An exciting morning's birdwatching indeed.

I go back for the great northern diver, locate it on my own, probably the same bird, fishing closer to shore this time. I sit and watch it with my ordinary binoculars. Back in my room I'm inspired to make a copy from a book-plate of this most beautiful bird, my sole attempt at bird illustration at art school. I'm no Robert Gillmor, though I still don't know who I am.

15. Drawing trips

Ray Atkins has come down to Falmouth, the same Ray from Reading. He's at last got himself a job teaching painting and is well pleased. Ray wants to get out and see Cornwall like me: the coasts and moors, the wild north coast and West Penwith peninsula, china clay mountains at St Austell, relics of tin mines at Redruth, the secretive wooded Fal and Helston rivers. And he has a van.

I ask him if he'll come along birdwatching in his van, see some of these places that way. Reaching bird sites by public transport is a problem. Trains don't go there, buses take for ever, and then you have to get back at the end of the day. Birding by bus on your own isn't much fun. Ray says if it's good enough for the birds, it's good enough for him.

We go first to Marazion Marsh. Ray relishes the wide rushing skies of Penzance Bay. He sees it all in terms of paintings to be made. I remember his large industrial landscape paintings from Reading. Thick impasto, slabbed, thrown, piled onto the board. Dramatic, hectic stuff: Oscar Kokoschka, Frank Auerbach. He's going to do the same with this landscape. I'm more interested in what's to be found in the reeds. The marsh is a modest area of reed and pools by the road, close to the tourist Mecca of St Michael's Mount, and also one of the star bird places of the county according to my well-used copy of John Gooders' *Where to Watch Birds*. 'Anything can, and does, turn up here,' says Gooders, magical lines for a birdwatcher.

I write: *Really good day out with Ray. Close views, the birds just there, no chases. Grey plover, sanderling and dunlin, ringed plover, curlew, redshank. Snipe in the marsh. We had great views of two seals rolling and playing in the breakers just off the beach. Curious of us, they came out of the water only five yards away to stare. Big mournful brown eyes and white whiskers.*

Not so many birds in fact for such a birding heaven, no rarities – it's often the case with the special place: the birds aren't there when you are. Or they're too far away, or it's just too cold and I don't hang around. I'm actually quite a bad birdwatcher, not a chaser or a twitcher, and easily distracted from the quarry. Though, with my new life-list, and adding new Cornish birds to it all the time, I can see that I might have developed into a twitcher. The term 'twitcher' as described by Mark Cocker in *Birders*, his great exposition of compulsive birdwatching, was first used to describe the shaking shivering half-dead birder in a motorbike sidecar arriving at the location of some rarity in dead of winter. My birding is about the unknown, the unexpected, going out there and just never knowing what you will find.

The college has a new minibus, and Ray has an idea to start up a weekly drawing trip for anyone who wants to go out for the day. I jump at it. He fixes it up and a few of us take off in the brand-new white Volkswagen. We drive to the dunes at Hayle in St Ives Bay, stay there all day crouched among the dunes and marram grass – at one with nature, you could say, or battling with it. Ray is in his element. Out in the sun and wind, under the great changing sky. I find him to be an immensely inspiring person to work with. It's a liberation for me. I forget myself, am absorbed into the great challenge of being outside, a part of all this. I draw at speed in charcoal on full A1 sheets pinned to a board. I pin a sheet of polythene to the back so the paper can be quickly covered if it rains. I don't know whether the work comes to anything but I get back to the minibus windblown, exhilarated. We drive home to the 'soft south', secluded Falmouth with its palm trees and tender gardens.

Next week we are on the Lizard peninsula (nothing soft about it), drawing the radio telescopes on Goonhilly Downs.

The great white dishes pointed at the sky are like something out of H.G. Wells. I get hold of these saucers, bright against a stormy sky, anchor them to the land. Again it's an exhilarating experience to be out in the elements all day, spurred on by them, carried into a near hallucinatory state by the wind; it's a state that somehow opens you up and allows the subconscious to take over. Ray, I can see, is doing the same. He works himself into a trance, scribbling and jabbing at the paper with oil pastels, smearing and blending with turps. I keep to charcoal and eraser, and white chalk to help bring it back 'up'. I fix the vulnerable charcoal with a spray that smells deliciously of pear drops. Ray is full of praise for my drawing – don't we all just need a bit of unconditional praise.

That evening, high on the fresh air and my drawing, I go up to the Summerhill, the art school pub at the top of Jacob's Ladder. I'll find some company, or company will find me. Maybe Lizzie from today's trip will be in tonight. Simon is often there. Ray doesn't go to the pub – he doesn't drink – but there are some regulars among the staff.

Andrew is one of them and drinking at the bar. 'D'you realise, when we're gone no one will remember *any* of this work of ours?' he cheerfully greets me. It's his pet subject, this gloomy existential prediction that even the best of us, the most successful students, are unlikely to ever be heard of in the future. Andy is pretty successful himself, a postgrad from the Royal College with his first lectureship at Falmouth, but he's sure that his name won't appear on any future score sheet. 'We won't even make a footnote in history,' he laughs into his beer, wiping his rather lush moustache.

Yes, I've finally broken in on the pub scene. Now that I'm here I'm as sociable and garrulous as anyone. I have this introvert/ extravert thing, not such an uncommon trait. But I do need a drink to bring out the extravert. I down pints of drink, euphoric.

Get myself oiled, plastered, pissed as a newt, and stay till closing time. Then I tackle Jacob's Ladder, reach the bottom in one piece, and go for a takeaway in the market square. Wind my way home along the main street with sausage and chips, some *Windy Night Rhapsody* playing through my head. The street held in a lunar synthesis. The street lamps sputter and mutter. The cat's in the gutter devouring a morsel of rancid butter. While *La lune ne garde aucune rancune.* Alone, I reach my front door, struggle with the key, find my small empty bed, last twist of the knife.

What privilege, art school! Etching, lithography, screenprinting, photography, film, ceramics laid on for you. In pottery, you can learn to throw on the wheel, be taken through the biscuit-firing, glazing and final firing of a finished pot; you can make a bowl, plate, jug, cup with handle, tea pot with a spout, handle and lid. There's a whole world of sculpture I hardly touch upon. And here we all are with our local authority grants, *paid* to be here. To experiment, try everything out, find what most interests us, and all without the need to come up with anything to show for it, or at least not much. To have made the exploration is justification enough. Oh it is rather *loose*, I suppose. A freedom that wouldn't pass now. I mean it's hardly value for money, is it?

As a painter I spend most of my time in the world of painting (and of course there are separate worlds within this). But I walk round with an art school camera in my bag too, take all the pictures I want, develop and print them as I go. And I take my drawing of the radio telescopes at Goonhilly Downs to the print room to make an etching from it. Then an aquatint. Welsh Gareth teaches me the processes: etching, where the acid eats into the lines you have drawn; aquatint, where the acid gouges areas of tone. I take to it right away and plan to do more. A notebook has a list of my future etchings of woods, sea and sky. It avoids the colour issue for one thing. It's all about tone and texture.

I'm interested in lithography too and plan my first lithos ... But after this term I don't get back to the print room. It burnt down. The place caught fire one night – almost certainly a student's cigarette – and burnt to a cinder. The chemicals stored there created such terrific heat, we came into college in the morning to find contortions of melted steel, girders bent like plasticine. By the time the place had been finally rebuilt, I'd moved on to pottery and ceramics. Then I made a film and I wouldn't get back to printing in my three years.

Gareth hears that I play classical guitar and employs me to teach his son the rudiments for some useful cash. He has also put me in contact with third year Ron, who is a more serious musician than me. Ron owns a fine and very expensive guitar – his singlemindedness in managing to acquire such a fabulous instrument is impressive. We work together on a transcription of the William Lawes *Suite* for two guitars, meeting every week for the rest of the year until he leaves. And our duet is a fine thing when it works, the chime of the two guitars greater than the sum of their parts, and a whole lot better than playing by yourself. Painting, of course, is very much a solitary activity. You follow your own path, dig your individual furrow ever deeper.

We painters have been encouraged to make our own stretchers for our canvases from the start. This is economical, good practice for the future. In the well-equipped carpentry workshop, we learn how to make a mortice and tenon stretcher joint, and bevel one side so the taut canvas doesn't rest on the wood. Canvas is cheap and off the roll. We learn to size it with rabbit skin glue. The brown 'rabbit skin', like a slab of toffee, is cooked up in a pan and brushed on the canvas while still warm. You can then lay on a thicker oil ground in white or a colour, or more easily work directly on the natural sized canvas. I find I can get free offcuts of board in the workshop and start to paint on these too – you can skip the rabbit skin glue stage with boards. Later, following Braque, I will pour sand into the primer to create a thick sandy ground. With oil painting, you paint 'fat over lean', using a higher ratio of oil to pigment as you go along, otherwise the paint surface will tend to crack in the future.

Ray appreciates all this 'free' material too, after years of struggling as an artist out there in the real world. I find him in the workshop making up his painting boards. He paints so thickly he needs the rigidity of hardboard and plywood rather than canvas. When he brings his work down from Reading, he rents a garage, 'the lock-up', to store them. This happens to be just opposite where I live in Swanpool Street and I help him unload. Heavy paintings! The crusty oil paint must have taken months to dry. Yet he packs them away with tenderness and care, with chocks and wedges so they don't damage each other, and swings down the metal door. 'The salt down here won't help', he says. 'It's the snag with art,' he laughs. 'Got to carry the bloody things around with you! Look after them, more and more of them. They're hard to sell,' he adds seriously, and explains his pricing method 'by the square foot'. The bigger it is, the more paint, the more it costs.

Ray's pictures seem so urban to me: waste ground, edge of town industrial sites, with great dramatic skies. Many are from Reading, I suppose. I remember he told me how nothing was finer to his eyes than a sunset through the smoking chimneys of some factory – the Port Talbot steelworks as seen from the M4 at sunset, for example.

'What about here, all these clean Atlantic skies?' I say, uneasy about this revelling in pollution merely for its colour effects, the ecologist and nature lover in me coming to the fore.

'What about Turner's *Rain, Steam and Speed*?' he replies. 'Turner loved a bit of industrial smog. Where shall we go for our next drawing trip?'

We drive inland to Ponsanooth Wood. This place is exciting

in a different way. It feels like a part of mysterious ancient Cornwall. The wood is wild, very dark, thick with ferns, filled with moss, encrusted with lichen. It feels remote, yet is only a few miles from the coast. It seems that no one ever comes in here. We clamber over barbed wire, push through a tangle of bush and brush, crush early wild garlic. In the heart of the wood there are ruins, perhaps of a mill, beside a boulder-filled stream. A magical place, a lost place – there's even a still, dark lake (water-filled quarry). Every surface of rock and tree is covered, shaggy, festooned with moss and lichen in the green gloom. The stream is placid now, just a chuckle, but we see by the tumble of boulders how it can rise to a torrent.

We separate with our boards and kit for the rest of the day. I work from the lane outside the wood, looking into its depths in the sunshine. Winter trees again. The dark tangle of Ponsanooth Wood in thick charcoal is my most successful Falmouth drawing to date, and much down to Ray's encouragement and enthusiasm. I love the place too, and will go back to live there in my third year.

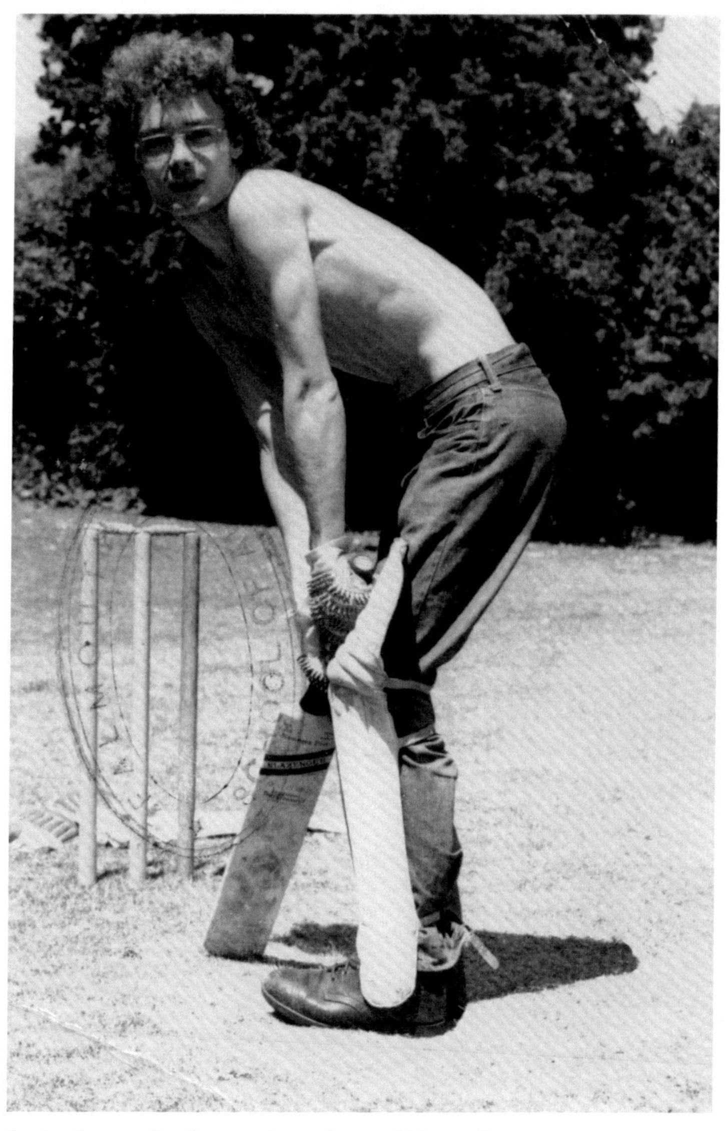

Invitation to the degree show dance, Falmouth 1977

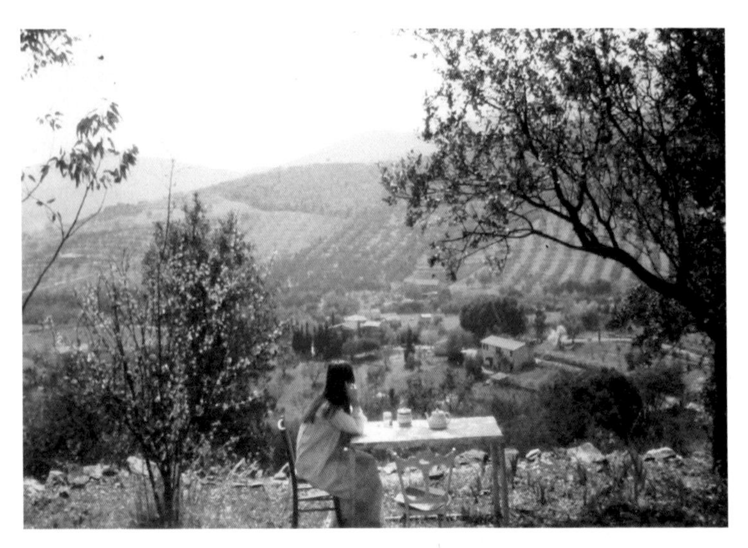

On the terrace at Porto Ercole

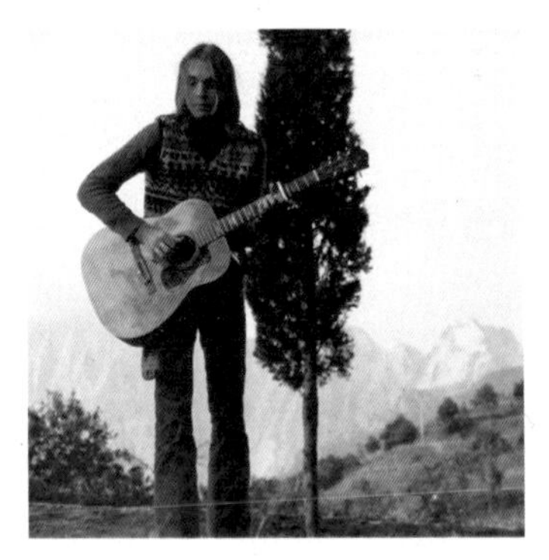

Mark Fry in Italy, 1971

(© Giorgio Cipriani)

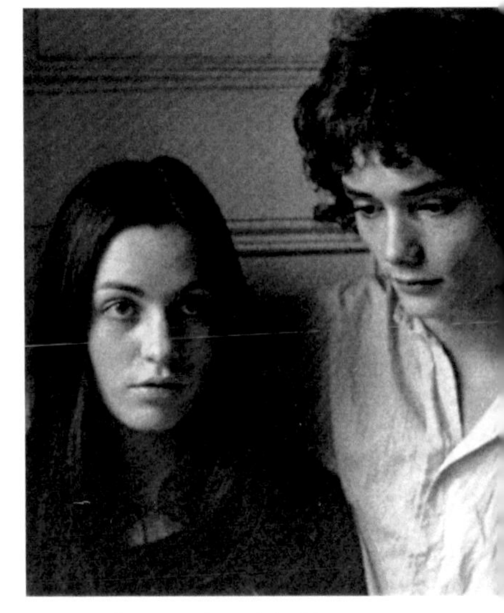

Home from Italy with Lise

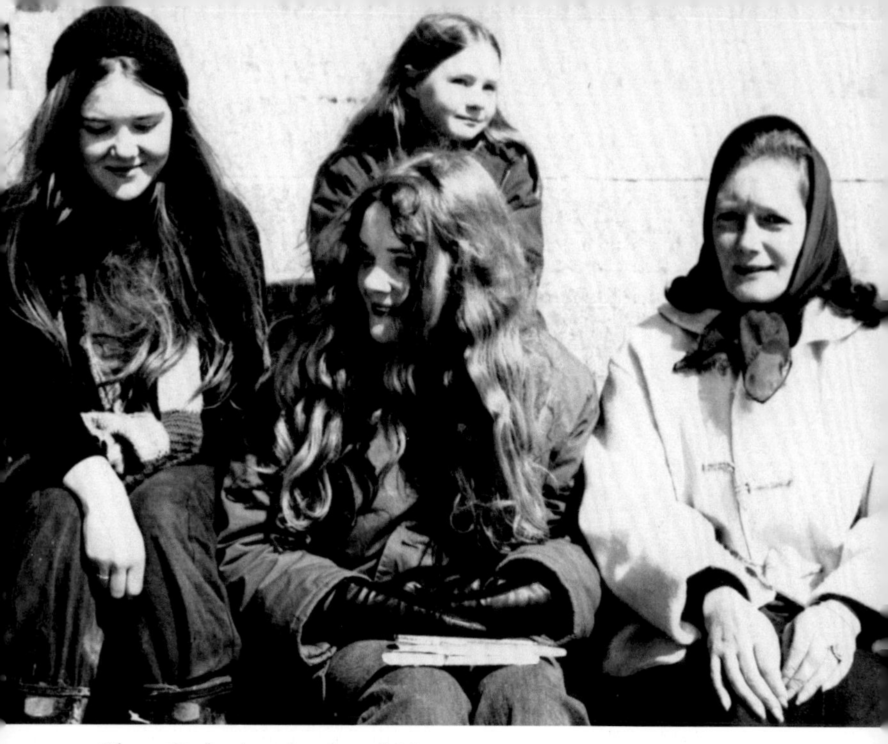

Clare, Catherine, Sarah and Mum

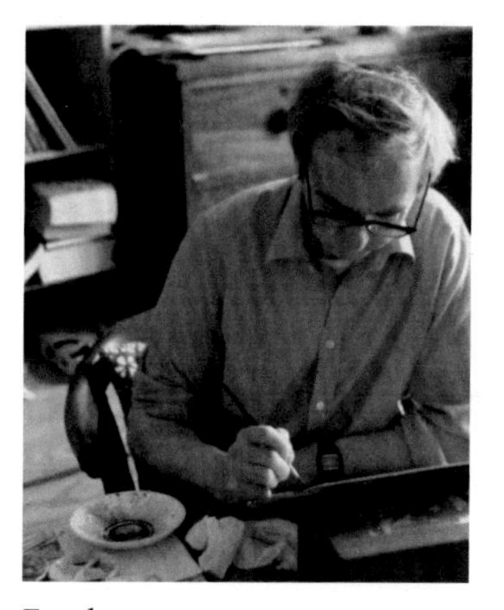

Frank

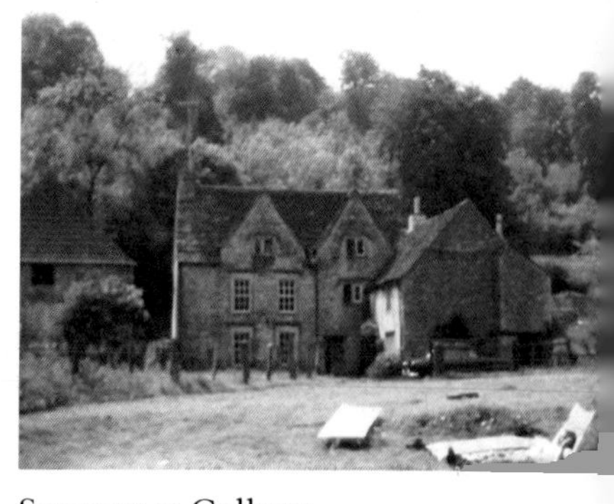

Summer at Colham

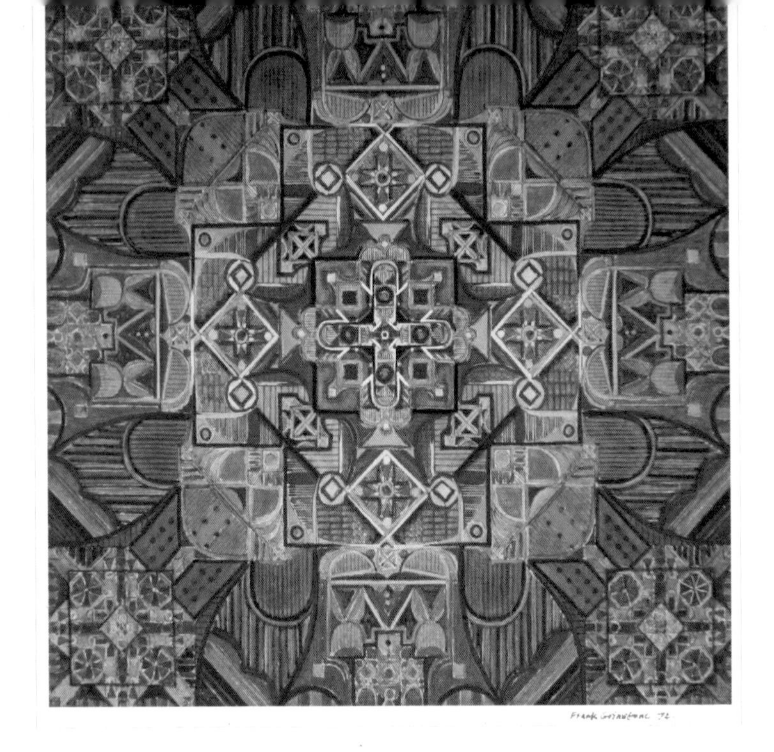

Frank's *Small Blue Abstract*

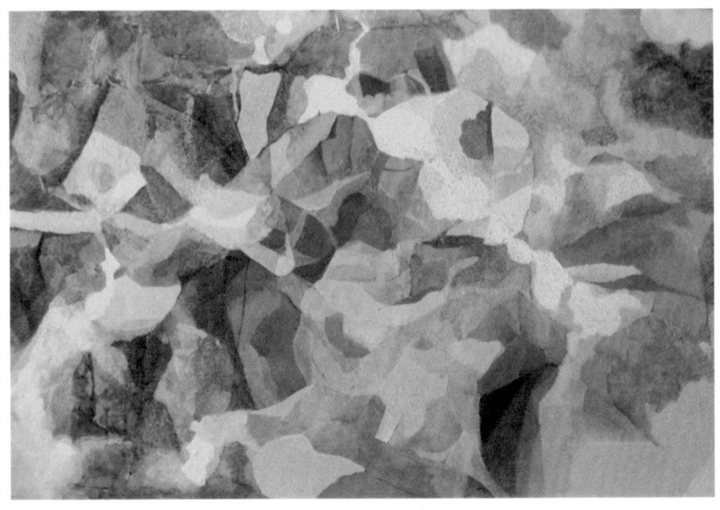

Dad's *Long Colham Landscape* (detail)

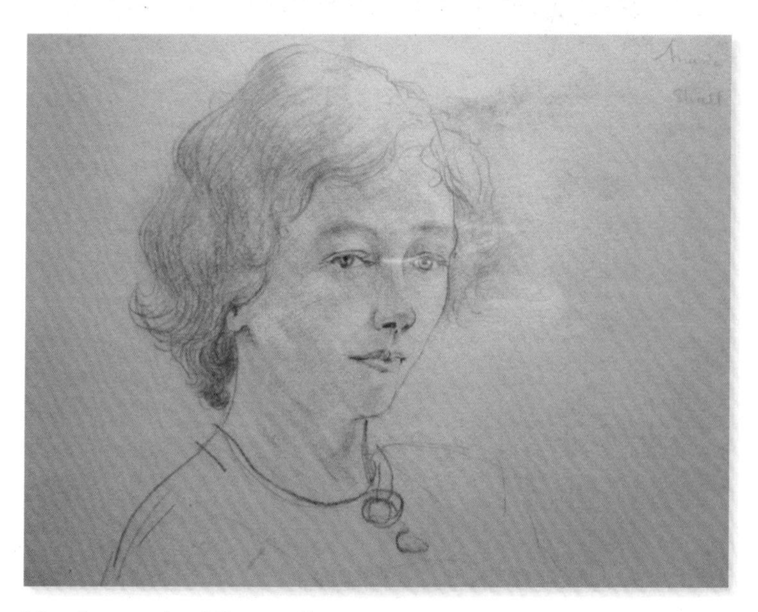

Mum's portrait of Granny Betty

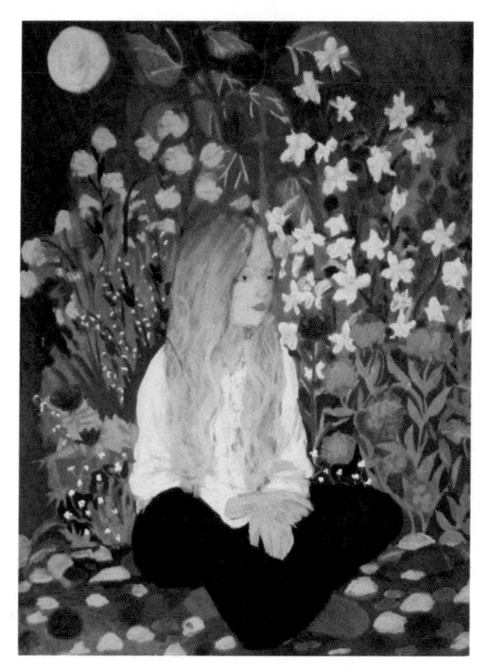

Clare's school painting of Catherine

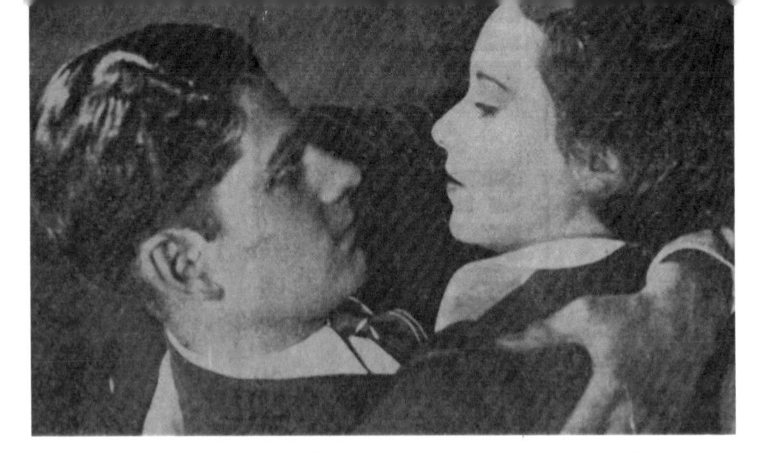

Helen Spencer (Granny Helen) and Laurence Olivier in *The Rats of Norway*, 1933

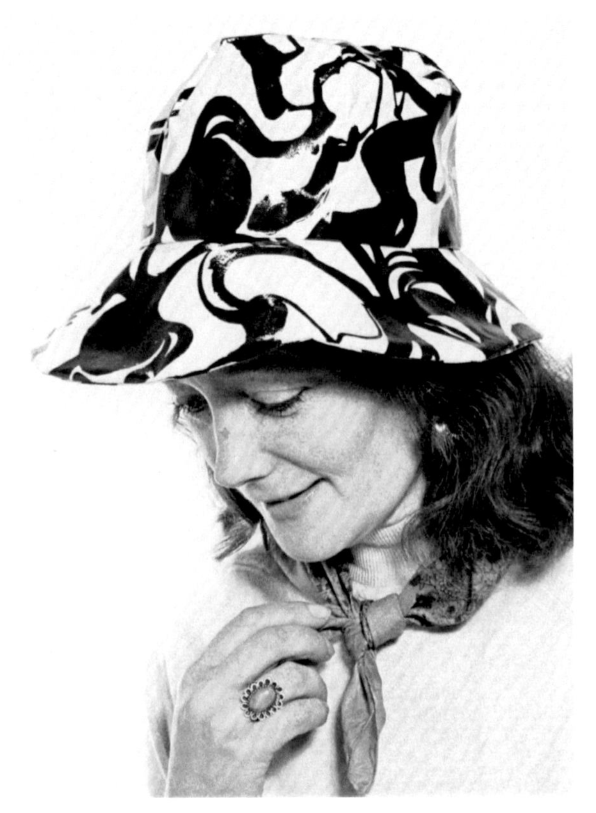

Mum portrait by Frank

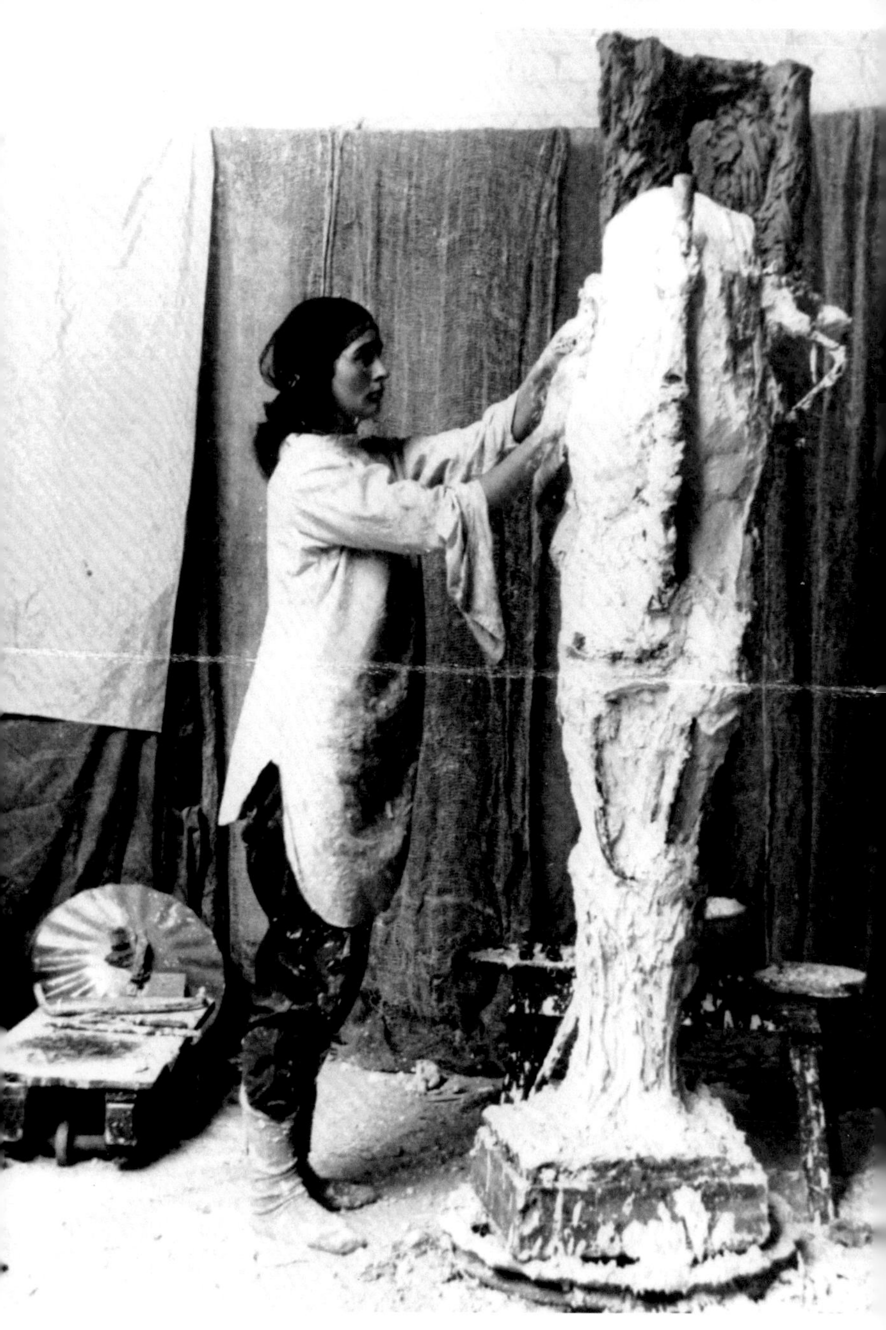

Corinne and her *Standing Figure*, *c.* 1958

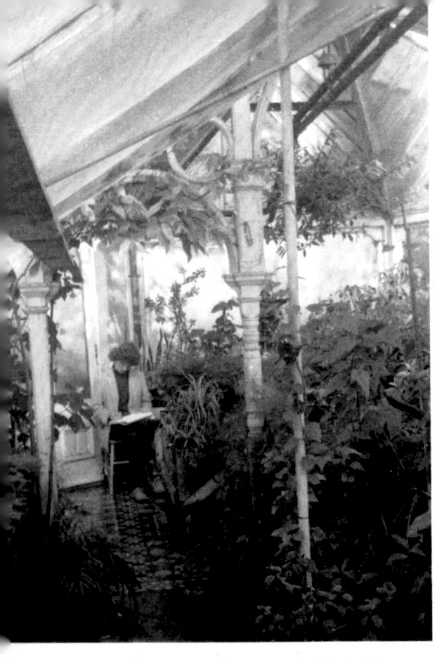

In the greenhouse at Reading
(© Jane Farrell)

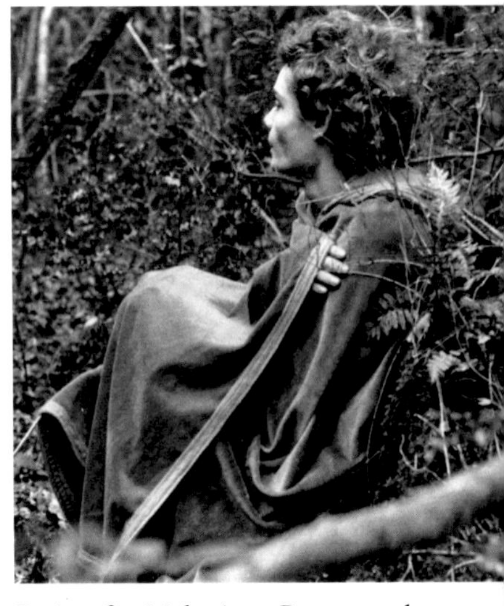

Posing for Melanie at Ponsanooth

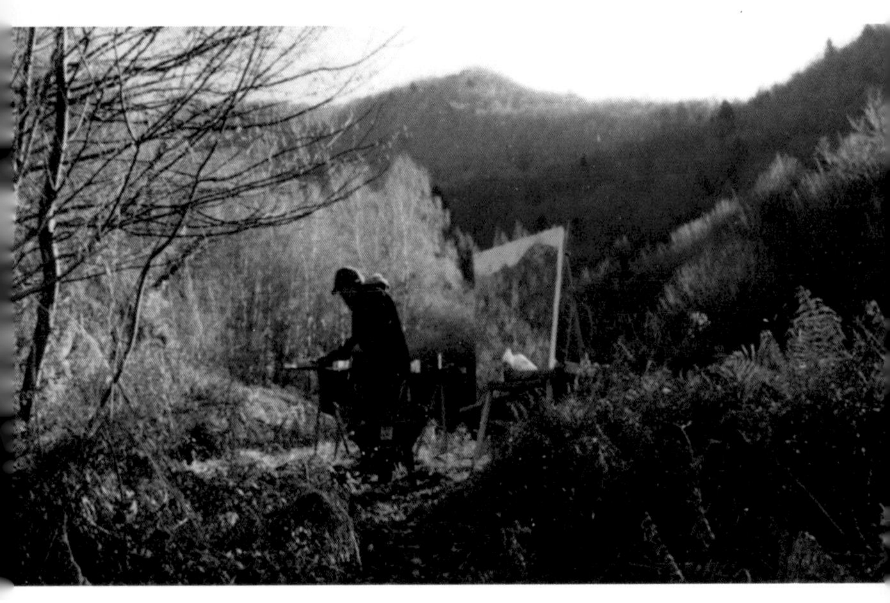

Ray at work *plein air* (© Ray Atkins)

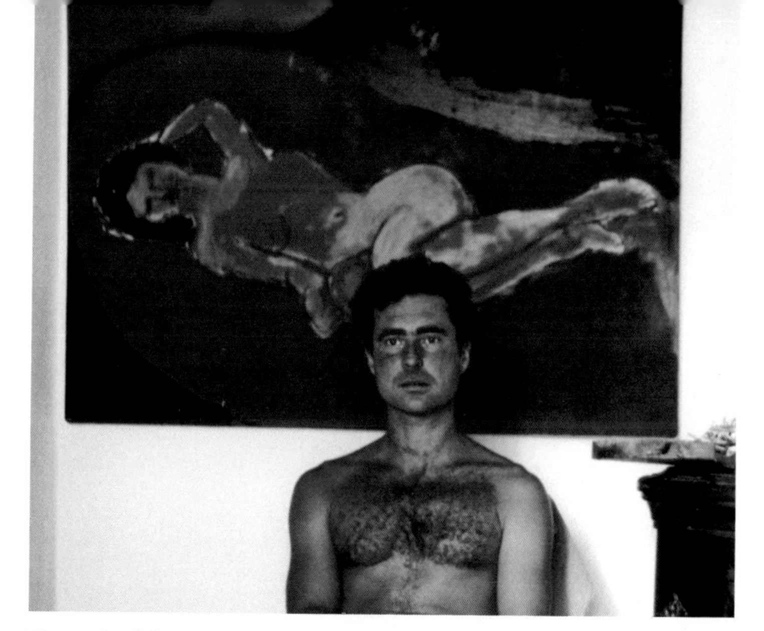

Simon in Alba

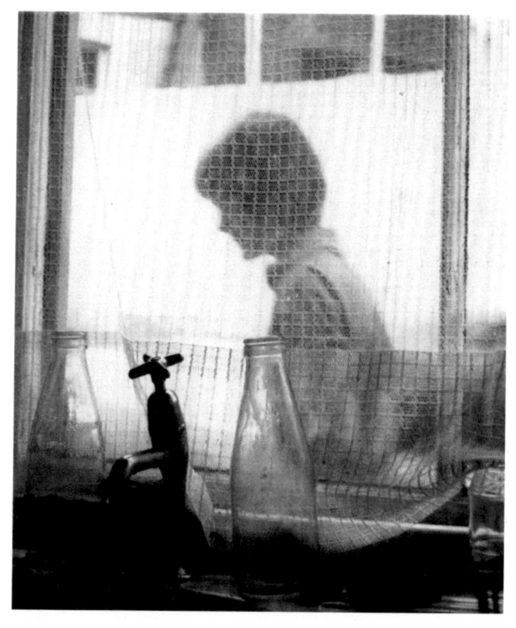

Kate outside the Swanpool Street kitchen

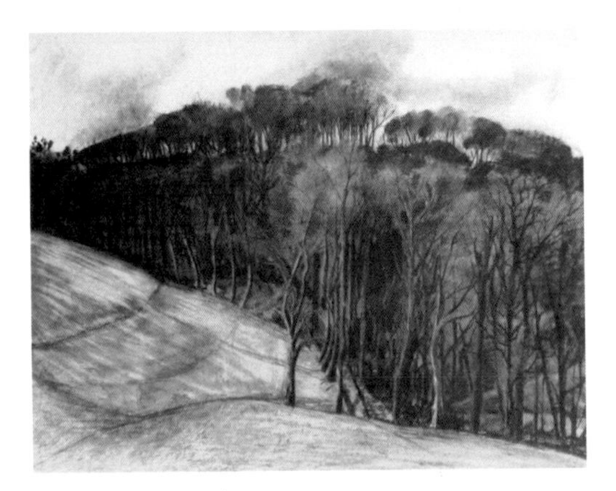

Ponsanooth Wood

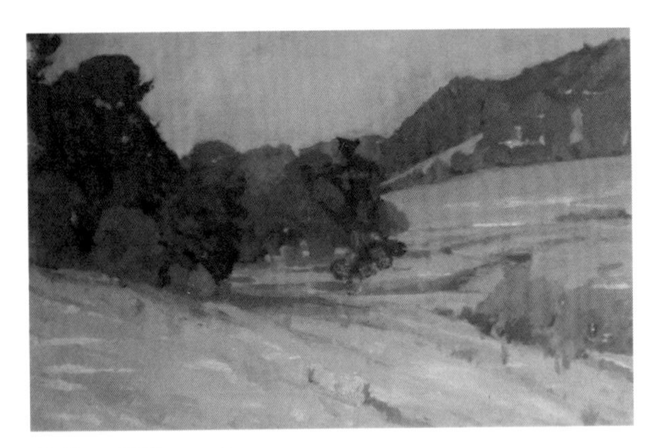

Colham Valley 1976

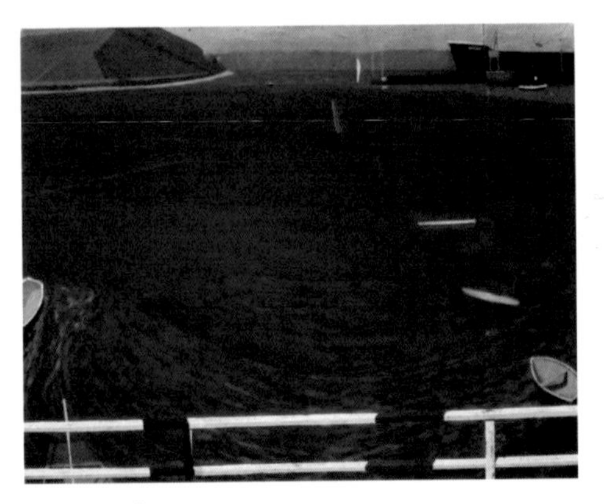

Blue Harbour

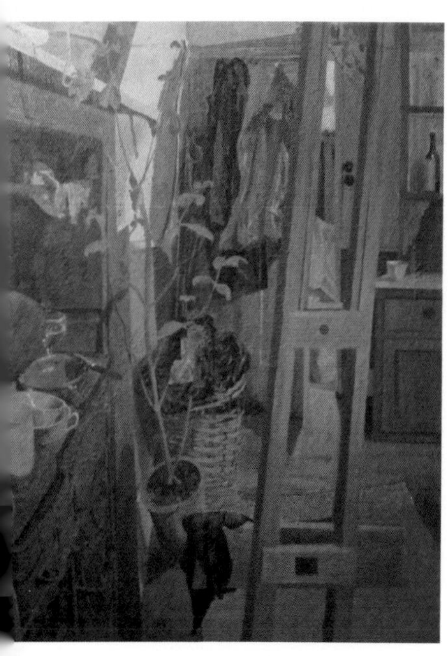

Swanpool Street Interior 3
(Stowell's)

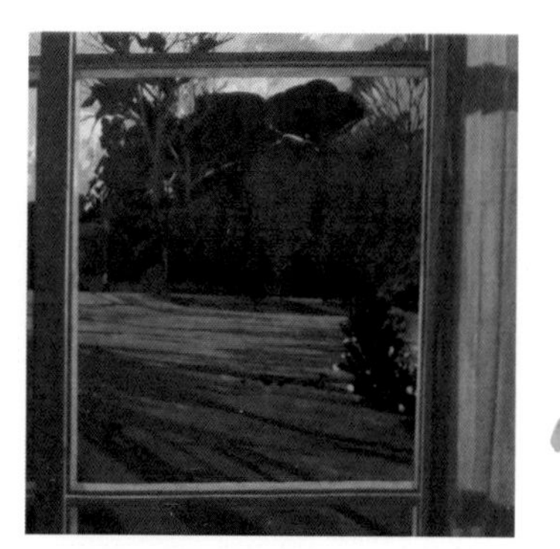

Window (funny greens
painting)

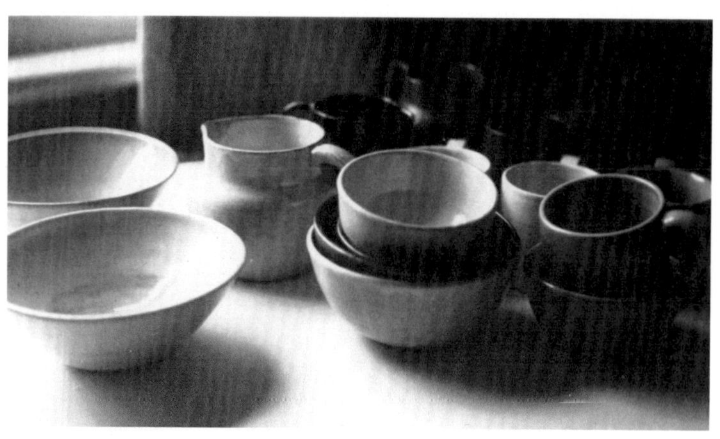

The set of pots

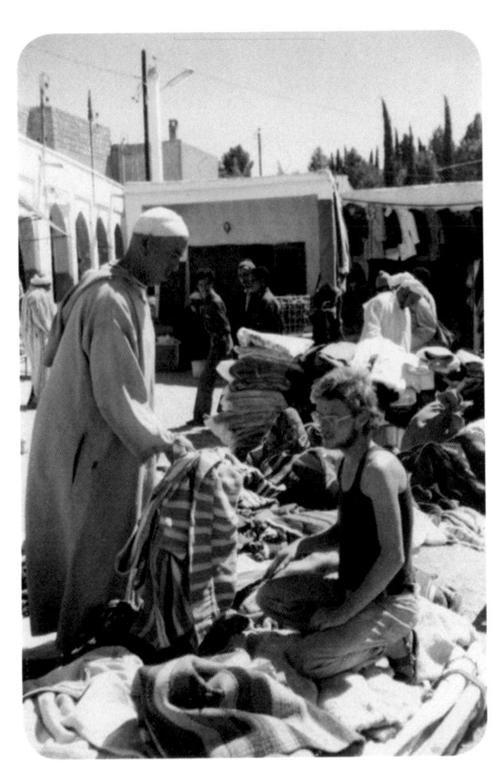

The trip to Morocco

16. Scilly Isles

In May I take a week out of college and go to the Scilly Isles. I don't tell anyone except Mrs Birch. A visit to these islands has been at the back of my mind ever since I knew I was coming to live in Cornwall – I talked about it with Granny. Granny can hardly get beyond her dustbins these days but she'll talk to you about getting to islands until the cows come home. The weather is fine and dry and looks like it might last. I quickly pack a tent, sleeping bag, primus, paints, notebook and binoculars, and get down to Penzance to board *The Scillonian.* The Scillies lie beyond Land's End, the furthest south-west point of England. There's something about geographical extremities with me. I will later be drawn to two of the most westerly points of Europe, the Blasket Islands, Ireland and Cabo da Roca, Portugal.

The ferry comes into the small harbour on the main island of St Mary's – 'Harold and Mary's island,' Granny tutted when the Labour Prime Minister retired here. I immediately see the pure white gull I was looking for, strutting about the quay. It has taken up occupation of the harbour and can be easily approached. My second Iceland gull this year. A good start. I take another boat out to one of the smaller islands, edge-of-the-world St Agnes, last stop before Bishop Rock. There are no cars on St Agnes. The campsite is a field beside the sea. There's a tap and nothing else. I stay for a week of almost unbroken sun and wind that tans my fair skin terracotta. I watch birds and beachcomb, fill a sketchpad with watercolours. These on-the-spot, unselfconscious sketches seem fresh and good to me, but they don't strike others that way. No one thinks much of them at all; they don't appreciate my sense of colour.

The birding is great, if weird at times. There are plenty of birds and birdwatchers around as it's the peak of the spring migration. I come across a crowd of them encircling a shrub which purports to contain a rare yellow-browed warbler – and am pleased to duly add the tick to my life list, while being conscious of the absurdity of the situation, grown men and women (mostly men) gathered in silence around a bush. People who have spent a lot of time and money trekking out here in order to do just this. Then they all troop off to the next bird, probably on another island. I stay put in my corner of St Agnes, with the gorse hedge brilliant yellow, the skylarks high in a blue sky, the horizontal lines of blue and green sea, white breakers, brown rocks. I move quietly, binoculars poised, along the narrow grassy lanes between fuchsia and honeysuckle hedges looking for more passerines.

I think about Granny. Picture her here, complaining loudly, yet probably happy enough. We talk about my island dreams, of being an RSPB warden on the bird islands of Skomer or Skokholm in Pembrokeshire, or why not here on the Scillies? And she tells me about her dream island, which is a pretty standard tropical one with everything tickety-boo and no mosquitoes. Where she would have all the time in the world to read *War and Peace*. In my tent, I brew up tea. Granny could be making her way round to tea at Waterloo Road about now. I remember a teatime a year ago.

Half past four. The family – Frank, Clare, Catherine, Sarah and I – gathered round the small deal table. Mum was missing. She was avoiding tea today by staying in bed; she was tired, that's true, but it was also easier not to come down and talk to her mother. Granny hadn't arrived from next door yet – 'I may be some time,' she quipped each day about this journey. There was a fresh white split-tin loaf, which Frank sliced evenly and thinly, and a fresh jar of Frank-made jam. I'd made the tea, put the cosy on the pot, and remembered the strainer.

After a while Frank said 'Has Granny actually been called?'

She hadn't. Clare, helpful as always, went round to fetch her. Granny had to see another human being at least once in her long fuddled day. She needed to see her daughter, Anne, even if they did end up fighting, and tea was the simplest meal to have with us – but she was sometimes forgotten. After the school day people didn't really have the energy for her.

I glanced at the clock on the wall out of habit. 4.35. The chink of cup on saucer, clatter of knife on plate seemed magnified in the crowded kitchen, as though through freshly-syringed ears. Catherine gobbled her bread and jam, gulped her tea. She had a new boyfriend, maybe her first real boyfriend, and was seeing him tonight. She had to wash her hair, and anyway she couldn't think of a thing to say to her loopy family. She wanted to get the hell out of the 'atmosphere' that descended at mealtimes, especially at tea. When I was seventeen I could never think of anything to say either.

Below the clock, Mum's painting of a Siamese cat with intense blue eyes. She did this amazing study of a cat's head before any of her four children were born, when she was seventeen and all set to become a star at Brighton Art School. When Granny, who posed for portraits by her talented daughter, was still a Brighton belle, as Frank put it. The painting was an inspiration and reassurance to me, and competition.

Little Sarah finished first. She beat Catherine and got out before her strange gran arrived. Granny had only come into Sarah's life a few years ago – suddenly appeared in the house and lived upstairs, crammed into Clare's old bedroom, turning the whole place upside down before they finally managed to move her next door. Now Catherine tried to melt quietly away too, but there was a kerfuffle at the door, where she collided with Clare and Granny coming in.

Granny was all in a fluster. She'd lost a bag containing some papers and money. We knew the bag wasn't lost, it was somewhere in her flat, and even if it was lost it wouldn't really matter. But she wouldn't rest until she found that bag, poor Granny. Frank would go round later and discover it in the fridge.

But her troubles could be put on the burner for now. She'd come to tea with her family, hair combed, her opal brooch on. She was wanted, even if half the young ones had left the table already and their mother not come down.

'Anne not here today?' she remarked.

'She's got a headache.'

'Always something.'

'It's just a headache, Granny!'

Frank stood up with a loud scrape of his chair and took his cup and plate out to the scullery. He checked the fridge for supper, which he would soon be cooking.

Granny prodded at her bread and jam, raised the large tea cup slowly, trembling, to her lips. We watched it return with a little rattle to its saucer.

'Must get on,' said Clare. 'You know I'm hoping to go to the *Slade*, Granny?'

'Oh yes, your mother went there after Brighton. She was such a clever girl.'

Clare was putting together her portfolio for her Slade interview. It was enviably large – paintings, pottery, embroidery, photographs, slides; the results of two fabulously productive foundation years at Taunton Art School – far more than I would take to Falmouth. I was left alone in the kitchen with Granny.

'Didn't get the wardening job on Skokholm Island in the end,' I said.

'Never mind. You did ospreys.'

How different she was from my other grandma in France. And while Frank called her a Brighton belle and got a laugh, she talked seriously about the years of scrimping, taking in ironing, scrubbing to the bone, just to make ends meet, 'to keep us all from the workhouse'. Fear of the workhouse was real for Betty in the 30s. It was a tough life in Rottingdean with her husband Teddy so often out of work, and fortunate in that respect that Mum was their only child.

I was ready to go with her to an island today in our conversation.

'You went to those Scilly Islands ... ' she began, mind-reading.

'Going, Granny. Going. And you can come too.'

'Yes! We'd need a rowing boat,' she said. 'And take Rags with us.'

Their dog Rags died nearly forty years ago, when Mum was still in her teens. I said, 'We'll take the ferry out there first, load up with provisions in the harbour of the main island, then go to one of the smaller islands from there. It needs to be quite a large boat.'

'Very large. You want good oars.'

'We can both row ...'

Of course it was about the island she already lived on next door at 69A Waterloo Road. It was always about getting away from there. Getting back to Rottingdean. She shouldn't have come here in the first place, should have been allowed to hang on in her home. We all realised that now. She didn't have any friends in Wellington. They were all back there dying, leaving her.

She was reaching for her stick, asking if she could see Mum now.

'Shall I go directly up?'

Exit Granny, hobbling up the hall, hobbling harder now she was about to see her daughter. She was thwarted, living here. Humbled by her dependence on the situation, on Frank. Her fierce old independence, her tattered pride battled every day with her situation, her deal of the cards. Was she intruding by going upstairs? Would Frank be cross? Wouldn't he have preferred her to go straight back to her bed after tea? He'd called her the most selfish person alive the other day. He could be so rude sometimes.

Tea was over. The table was only half cleared. People had taken their cup and plate out to the scullery but left most things as usual. In a way it wasn't worth clearing the table as supper was a mere hour and a half away – there were so many meals in a day at home. Granny would have her supper taken round on a tray.

The kitchen went quiet. Frank was at the back room table going through a master game of chess from a book in this small window of free time. Upstairs the water pipes gurgled as Catherine washed and conditioned her golden curls. Clare was in the attic with her portfolio. Sarah was on the sitting-room floor watching *The Virginian*, mouthing her homework aloud. And Mum, drugged and half asleep in bed with her migraine, was unaware that her mother had begun creeping up the stairs.

Down on my Scilly island beach, I spot a lesser yellowlegs, a scarce vagrant, which has been blown across from North America. It isn't difficult to see – it's just a redshank with yellow legs – and only a matter of being in the right place at the right time. I think about this rarity business, which seems to me to be the whole basis for twitching. The lesser yellowlegs is a common wader in the States. Why not just go and see it there? Not that I didn't I enjoy spotting it by chance, making the identification. And it was good to see the yellow-browed warbler – I felt for it, blown off course from the Siberian taiga with no chance of ever getting back there, ever finding a mate; a doomed bird. I noted its small differences from the other leaf warblers: pale yellow band above black eye stripe, and so on. The wonder of diversity is definitely for me. It's just this mad pursuit of the hapless blown-off-course creature that seems all wrong.

But there are birds, ordinary birds, everywhere on the islands this week. Beach, sea, field and scrub are alive with them – you hardly have to look. There are fresh falls of migrants daily and it's a joy to be among them. I visit some other islands, see interesting birds on the small grassy airfield of St Mary's, among the pools of the garden island of Tresco. I visit the gardens of Tresco for Mrs Birch in a way – half the plants in her garden seem to come from here; her marvellous echium spike is from a seed 'smuggled out'. Some of the resident birds seem to be almost tame, as though they have nothing to fear. I invite a song thrush into my tent to pick up morsels of cheese, photograph it beside my Doc Marten boot. It cocks its head and eyes me, wise thrush. I lie on my back on the grass and watch the skylarks rise and fall in the summer sky.

Yes, it's a wonderful place to be. A small-scale place, with small hedged fields for the early daffodils, small lanes that take no cars, small buildings hunkered down out of the wind. What a safe place it is. There surely is nothing to be frightened of here.

'You had a good time then,' grins John from Dartmouth in the canteen queue, referring to the livid colour of my face after a week of sun and wind. Tan as much as you can, is the mantra we all follow. Skin cancer, what's that? We blithely lie out in the midday sun. There are no other remarks about my week's absence from college. Has anyone even noticed? But I've done enough work to justify my trip anyway. I scan the occupied tables in the canteen, wonder which one to sit at, which one to try and join.

17. Drawn from life

For *Swanpool Street Interior* 3 I prepare my 'Braque ground': plywood board nailed to a strong frame, primer mixed with sharp sand to produce a textured surface, and carry it home to my room – it weighs a ton. Then I just paint a corner of the room with the iron range and glass sideboard, the door ajar. Everything seems to work with this painting: the wine bottle placed just so, crockery on the range, pot plant weaving across the picture surface. I put in the easel I'm working on, right up on the surface, the picture plane. The bold diagonal of the easel unifies it all. An easy painting to do, it doesn't take long. And it goes down well when I lug it into the studios to show Dick Platt. He wants to enter it for the Stowell's Prize.

I go back to the studios and the life room. Simon seems to be getting the most out of life drawing. He's always there, small and wiry, nervy, standing at his easel. Ray comes in too. Sometimes he runs the session but he ensures he does his own work as well. He's a furnace of energy which blows across the room to me. You can hardly see which is landscape and which is figure with his work. I persevere, drawing Suzanne and others, sometimes a male model too. I'm working finely in pencil again, trying to discipline myself, looking at the anatomy books.

Hewlett comes into the studio one day to do a portrait of the model, clothed. He sweeps in with easel, paints and model. He hangs a brown cloth on the screen behind the model and arranges her. Arranges Suzanne's head, the angle, direction to light; raises her chin, adjusts it slightly to the left; refines the position gently with his hands like some beaky doctor. Then he places a small canvas on the easel, sketches the shape of the head and hair, and blocks in the background. He works swiftly from general down to detail: girl with orange hair against brown. It's fascinating to watch his hawklike intensity, his rapid manner of working. In an hour – perhaps that's all he's paid her for – he has finished, packed up and gone.

My pencil life drawings aren't working. I go back to rougher charcoal, which suits me better, which is more like landscape – the curves of form, the lights and shades. If I can just get as involved in the human body as I do with landscape, the shapes of woods and hills and clouds, the same principle of immersion. The model stays still, like the landscape, only the light moves. The body's curves are immensely subtle, but then so are a landscape's. But the feeling of oddness and artificiality remains. Working with the landscape I don't get this. It doesn't seem contrived like this. It's normal and right to be out there trying to render something of nature on the flat surface of paper or canvas.

By the end of my three years I'll be able to do a passable drawing of the figure, but it never takes off for me, never really gets beyond this student level. I don't have the passion for drawing the human body that Simon or Ray have. And as I've said before, I find the whole business of the clothed drawing the unclothed odd. Well, I just get too involved, I suppose, as I caress the paper with my stick of charcoal. Like Picasso et al, I'm a randy goat hot for my model, wanting some *après-atelier* relief. But my model goes home to her boyfriend after the day's work and I go back to my room, my still life painting, *nature morte*, as the French call it.

Down in the second and third year studios, the students have their own spaces where they can screen themselves off for privacy. There's a bit of a fetish about this hiding behind sheets and bedspreads from all prying eyes. No one's seeing inside my space. The star painter, Colin Smith – a tall swarthy Londoner with moist cow eyes and long lashes and a surprisingly small voice – is high on the secretive list. He works behind swathes of protective sheets. And he's always there, so it's hard to get a peep. A huge dark canvas, canoe shooting under a Thames bridge, the rowers bowed with exertion, their long oar blades cutting the water; thin, sloshy, dripping paint – quite Francis Bacon, it seems to me. You know Colin's the real thing, though; everything about him spells out painter – and his work is in collections all over the world now. In the next cubicle, also well-curtained, is his acolyte Tony, who also does these dark Baconish paintings – I remember horses in a brooding landscape. Right now I prefer their neighbour Crispin's work: an intense study of a snooker table, the player hunched over his cue, the bright-lit green baize; a very still painting of electric light and the night, which proceeds slowly. The eeriness of Edward Hopper comes to mind.

At the other end of the studios, another third year star. Skeet is an intense Scottish girl who is working on viewpoint and vision. She's producing this messy (very Euston Road) painting, which seems to take her for ever, of the studio seen from one fixed viewpoint, and I think one eye, as she always seems to have one closed or be wearing an eyepatch. It's all radiating lines from the viewer's eye, grubby with pencil marks, and does in a way rather resemble the paint-spattered studio floor, screens and bits of furniture. Skeet will get a First and go on to post-graduate at the Slade, her spiritual home.

There's a drawing trip with Ray to the china clay pits at St Austell, a rescue from the studios. On a grey sultry day we lose ourselves among mountains of clay waste. The new ones are dirty white, a lunar landscape. The older ones, at different stages of being colonised by vegetation, are oddly conical green mountains. The weird landscape suits my charcoal and chalk. In my mind's eye now the almost comical mountains mingle with my earliest pictures, done in Frank's studio that first summer I arrived at Waterloo Road aged seven, when Frank gave me some grey card and Conté chalks to draw my lunar mountains and craters. Hot and thirsty, calling to each other over the echoing clay hills, we reunite with our work of the day. As ever Ray is full of praises for my efforts. While I am astonished by his oil pastel drawing, a little envious of his extravagant colour additions to this essentially white and grey landscape.

Ray takes me to the site of his painting on the north coast, on the cliff tops at Portreath, near where he lives. Heavy plywood board, industrial-size paint cans, palette knives and spatulas, easel and guy ropes: some gear, all of it carried from the van. It's his first full-size painting, his real Cornish initiation, far out on the cliffs. 'A four-foot board for starters. The six-footer might have been trouble!' He complains about the wind. There's always a wind to contend with, he says, and it seems to double in strength as soon as we arrive. There are no straight lines here, only wobbly lines. It's a case of stab and see. One of the difficulties of course, I see, is just where you can set up on a scale like this; it doesn't necessarily correspond to where you wanted to be, your first vision of the place. You have to make do, go with the flow.

'Why don't you take photographs? Take them back to the studio,' I say.

Ray splutters. Of course he isn't the photographic sort. He has to be out here. Feel the air, the racket of gulls and crash of waves, smell of briny, whistle of the wind through the guy ropes. Woolly hat clamped to his head, eyes screwed into the wind. And of course I know all that. It's what I'm like, I'm finding out. You don't get long, he says. In these conditions you have to slam on the paint and go at it as fast as you can. Work with a symphony going through your head. And sometimes it works.

Kate comes to live at Swanpool Street for a short time, though oddly I have almost no memory of it. I know she's there but can't pin it down. She's not painting at all now; we don't get together to discuss work. I think she takes Charlotte's room – I hardly saw Charlotte after she left the house, but that was how it was; you quickly moved on to new people. Anyway, Kate was suddenly there and I took a photograph of her in the street through the kitchen window. I heard her leave the house and caught her as she turned up the hill, head slightly bowed, in silhouette through the lace curtain. I make an enlargement of it, keep it. There's so little there, a blurred shape through the curtain, but it's Kate.

I negotiate a decorating job with Mrs Birch in lieu of rent and seem to spend the rest of the summer painting her hall, stairs and landings. It's all a pale aquamarine gloss – walls, ceiling, woodwork. I paint it in gloss again. Heady job. Ingestion of CFC fumes for weeks. But no different from doing my father's hall and stairs in that dark brown gloss last summer. As I work, 10cc's passionate song 'I'm not in Love' is playing on the radio. Which is also the case with me.

Kate has gone now and Pasters has moved in. He's having a torrid affair with an American girl. One afternoon I wander into his room without knocking, or rather I knock and don't wait, and find them coupled on the bed. Two faces from another world turn to look at me. I apologise and flee.

Pasters is unfazed. 'No hard feelings, old chap. What a girl, though.' He keeps telling me about his fabulous American girlfriend, how much he's learning. The Brits, she says, don't know a thing about fucking. And it's true I don't even know about the position I witnessed. Sitting up.

'It's all the time, John. Time after time!' he says.

Such self-confidence is certainly something to aim for.

Pasters' super-optimism and unshakeable self-belief, both of which I desperately admire, remind me of De Gruyter. And bizarrely, another moment of accidental voyeurism along these lines occurs this summer.

I pay a visit to Reading for my year's Fine Art degree shows. There's Mud and Karen, Marg and Peter, Dee and Stephen. Dee is getting married soon. There's Pete Hay again, not seen since my goodbyes to Lise on Reading Station. I would like to seek out my old girlfriend Mandy, but that's long over and done with. I go round the exhibitions, am amazed by the professionalism of my old colleagues' presentation of themselves in a finished show. De Gruyter gets a First, I note. Pete shows me his work and impresses me with his intense ink-and-watercolour landscapes that have hardly changed since he first arrived; he has some stranger, darker collages too, after Baudelaire's *Les Fleurs du Mal*, which he made following a decadent trip to Amsterdam – a bunch of them went off there with Pete, like his trip to Wittenham Clumps; I'm envious of that. I won't see him again until 1986, when I come back to live in Reading and we become good friends. I have his paintings on my walls now.

But I'm an onlooker at the degree shows of '75, not part of this place any more. I wander round the old London Road site, unable to stick with anyone during the afternoon's drinking on the lawn. I don't see my father there, which is some relief. I miss a moment of drama when someone pours a pint of beer down a lecturer's back. There's still plenty of discontent with some of the lecturers. There has been a very high drop out in my year – a third of us never graduated. Years later I heard that Roger Cook had apologised for the level of the teaching, saying they hardly knew *how* to teach then.

Sidelined, drunk myself, I retreat up a fire escape – to look down on the proceedings perhaps, to smoke in peace – only to blunder into a couple making love at the top. Lise and De Gruyter! I turn the top corner of the iron steps and there they are. I don't know if they see me. I back down quietly, slip away, find somewhere else to feel left out. I must get back to Falmouth.

Someone's at the bathroom door, lurking on the creaky Swanpool Street landing. 'D'you have a drop of hot water for a shave?' Mrs Birch's father, the 'Colonel', proffering a tin mug. I help him half fill it from the explosive gas geyser. He won't shave in the bathroom but goes back to his room.

The Colonel has the room next to Pasters'. He has brought his dachshund with him, which makes at least four of the little yappers in the house. The old Colonel seems mad as a hatter to me, and that tightens me up. It's all a bit close to home.

He arrived in a state. Wrenched from his home. But he couldn't live alone at home any more, had to have someone look after him, and his daughter was really the only option. Father and daughter do not get on. They find fault, blame each other for everything. It is indeed another version of Granny Betty's kidnap from her beloved Rottingdean and imprisonment next door to her ogre daughter at Waterloo Road. Like Granny with her pipe dreams, the Colonel is always trying to get back to his house in distant East Anglia. One day he calls a taxi and reaches Exeter before the driver twigs. He is brought back to Falmouth humbled, and charged a hundred pounds.

He continues to make a nuisance of himself in the house. Writes to the Queen about his imprisonment and his 'stolen' medals. Pasters plays up to him with salutes, a bit of military barking. 'Ah, Colonel,' he blusters when they meet on the landing. 'How *is* it? How's the *leg* bearing up?' The old boy loves this and calls Pasters 'the Lieutenant'.

Like the Colonel, I have my grandfather Teddy's medals from the First World War. Granny Betty gave them along with Great Granddad's silver cup. I haven't sold these. I admire and treasure them. I wonder at the bravery that earned them. The array of medals with their bright ribbons are kept safely at home with my old coin collection.

A Mrs White, 'friend' of the Colonel, visits while I'm decorating. It's always awkward decorating staircases – a painter on the stairs seems to draw people out of their rooms. Suddenly, everyone has to be going up and down stairs, and I'm having to make room, move the ladder, mind the paint pots, while they squeeze past.

Mrs White emerges from the C.'s room and shrills down to the owner of the house, 'There's no toilet paper!'

'Everyone keeps their own in their room!' Mrs Birch calls back.

'Nonsense! You think people walk around with a toilet roll in their pockets? You expect me to arrive as a guest with my own? This is all most disorganised. What you need here is organisation. I've run a boarding house, you know. Fancy having the stairs repainted and no toilet paper.'

Mrs Birch is acting oddly. She has taken to coming upstairs a lot, suddenly appearing in the landing outside her father's room, muttering. She thinks they are hatching plans in there: Mrs White is going to run off with him.

There's someone at the front door. An uproar of barking from the dachshunds but Mrs Birch isn't opening. I go. It's a cross young nurse for the Colonel. I show her up. My knock on his door is met with more ferocious barking from his sausage dog. Its owner comes to the door in assorted underwear, garters and braces. He looks haggard, there's a bruise on his face. I have to shout to tell him about his visitor who is standing right beside me. When he sees her his manner changes to one of utmost politeness and decorum.

With 'sitting-up' Lieutenant Pasters around it gets loud at Swanpool Street. Like De Gruyter he cultivates an entourage wherever he goes. People from Sculpture I don't know fill the kitchen. Big wheezy Derek with his handlebar moustache and his girl, Jill. Johnnie, the local boy from St Ives, who is also boldly moustached. They hang about, as does Dave, the boatbuilder from the attic, ever more shadowy, attaching himself to the group. Dave latches onto me, and I wish he wouldn't. He sees me as a soft touch. Certain lonely people always have, and in truth their neediness puts me right off. I'm really just as much hard nut as sensitive soul. 'Dave, I'm working! No time to chat!' I take my coffee back to my room. We all troop off to the pub on the waterfront and Dave sits with me. Oh I'm okay with Dave. I help him along, and he helps me in a way, makes me feel bolder, more of the group of which I am also on the edge.

In the life room I work alongside Irish Joseph. I don't have a woman to make love to like Pasters, but I can draw one with my pent-up frustration in thick smeary charcoal. Joseph seems to feel pretty much as I do about life drawing. He screws up sheets of paper in rage and despair. But the drawings anger him less than the fact that he's here drawing at all. The ivory tower nature of the art school is really getting to him now. 'Will you just look at what's happening now in the Bogside. What the *hell* am I doing down here in *lovelee* Cornwall? Wasting everyone's time, *am'nt I*?' he cries again. There's plenty of this from the bottom-of-my-heart wailing about the value in what we are doing. And what indeed is the value in it? A part of me is happy to agree that it's nothing at all. It isn't going to do anything for Derry anyway. It's like Auden's remark about poetry making nothing happen. Conscience-stricken Joseph eventually takes his turmoil to Northern Ireland to do a project and I don't remember him returning to finish the course.

I take a week off painting to do a joinery course in the workshop. We can make an object of our choice. I make a miniature chest of drawers like the one my father once gave me and I still use to keep treasures found on walks: pebbles, beach glass, fossils, feathers, fragments of birds' eggs. Using this as a template, copying the dovetail joints, I construct a chest of matching dimensions with eight drawers instead of six. It takes a week, and the drawers stick on their runners, but I oil and buff the wood and proudly stand it alongside the original.

I also make a pair of sandals in the workshop. An enthusiastic young Aussie gives a day's course in constructing everlasting sandals with car-tyre soles. It's a relief from too much Fine Art.

And I take to swimming. The English Channel, once expectations are lowered, becomes refreshing and tingling, and I aim for a daily dip.

My sister Catherine writes me a letter – a poem – descriptive of summer's night that waxes on for several pages in Romantic style. She doesn't say what she's doing but it's around the time she moves out of Waterloo Road for a while to stay on a farm with a girl friend. I know she wants to get out of the claustrophobic family house like me and Clare. I wonder why she won't be joining our father's summer camping holiday to France. I suppose it's all her decision, maybe to do with exams. Or has there been some other obstacle? She has completely changed her handwriting for this letter, imitating Clare's, which surprises and somehow disappoints me. Dad approves of it, thinks it a positive move, a kind of reinventing oneself. To me it seems more like a loss of part of your true self.

18. Summer holiday

I set off in my sandals to meet Clare in London. She has moved out of student hall and is sharing a flat above a shop in Kensal Rise with a film maker called Chris Welsby, a postgraduate at the Slade; his brother Richard, a painting student at Chelsea, is there too. It feels she's going up in the world. We link up with Dad and Catherine H's Peugeot at the ferry, then dawdle our way through France. Our father is something of a Francophile and over the years has travelled widely on its back roads. Which makes it even stranger that he's never been to see his mother in Biot. He was never invited, and I suppose he never asked. The original family ban on the children from Granny Helen's previous marriage laid down by wicked stepfather Tully held good for the rest of his life.

Neither Clare nor I can drive yet. We are kids in the back seat of our father's car as we meander south, stopping at cathedrals (the marvel of Chartres), the Loire, camping overnight in the Municipal, and ending up on a patch of waste ground near Estagel in the foothills of the Pyrenees. Just somewhere we can camp, flat ground by a river, rather than being a campsite per se. I get out my paints, my easel. Now I'm an art student with an artist father. We work *plein air*. Dad does a watercolour of the river through the poplar trees, the strip of water intensely blue, half of the paper left blank. I set up among the docks and thistles, work in oil on paper. The place is full of wildlife. *Plagues of flies and wasps. Stick insects, praying mantises, black shiny beetles with a scorpion tail, red crickets with blue wings, great green grasshoppers, cicadas. A million* grenouilles *croaking*. Dad sees a snake swimming across the river while he works: *ochre and sienna with a zig-zag stripe down its back*. There are many birds. I see an exotic hoopoe, and bee-eaters fly over with their lovely tinkling calls.

It's good to share my interest in birds with Catherine H. We visit the Étang de Canet, famous for its flocks of greater flamingo, and watch these stately creatures wading through the shallow pools. We track down fan-tailed warblers along the edge of the lagoon, and a possible aquatic warbler too, though this is outside its range. It's a bird-filled holiday. Sixteen black kites fly slowly in to roost by the camp one evening. On a memorable drive over the bare limestone plateau of Les Causses, we counted 29 raptors, most of which we failed to identify – as is still the case with me and distant unfamiliar birds of prey. Memorable too that day was acute food poisoning from a plate of mussels in a restaurant near Perpignan, my first such attack from rogue shellfish. The mussels tasted fine. You never can tell.

Then Clare gets ill, very ill. The doctor in Estagel says she's too ill to be camping. Dad fixes her up in a hotel in the town and we visit her every day. Her medication, it being France, is in the form of suppositories, which we English always find hard to swallow, so the family joke goes.

That night I lose my paints. I leave a wet oil painting on the easel overnight – 'Ah, sur le motif,' father intones, as though I were Paul Cézanne out at his Mont Sainte-Victoire, and I do feel proud – and next morning it's still there. On the ground. Easel and paint box have gone! The thief's discerning eye in leaving the painting behind becomes another family joke.

Already September. The others have set off on the slow drive home. Clare, recovered from her 'flu ('the worst I've ever had'), stays on with me and we hitch down to Spain together. Our route curiously re-enacts my first trip to Spain with Lise five years ago when I was so head over heels in love. This seems extraordinary now but at the time I was hardly aware of it, my singing out with joy when we ended up in places I'd already been to with my ex. Of course I don't have anyone now and

I imagine Clare doesn't either. She doesn't tell me that she got together with Richard, the guy sharing her flat, the very night before I arrived in London. She's waiting to see what will happen on her return, and as we hitch south into Spain, very close to each other, I recall, I'm kept unaware of Richard.

But as far as the replaying of my journey of teenage love goes, of course you can't do these things twice. It isn't the same. Clare and I have our own adventures, some of them quite uncomfortable, which overlay the other trip like more recent photographs. Our first stop is just over the border at Porto de la Selva – you could say it stands for nearby Cadaqués, the village visited with Lise, with Salvador Dalí's castle up on the cliffs. Here, I confidently lead Clare up the scrub hillside outside the port to pitch our little tent, and we are murdered in the night by the tiny mosquitoes. Next day, while we are nursing bites and puffy faces in the sea, a thunderstorm demolishes our tent, and we retreat, chastened, to the Municipal, which is perfectly okay and a much more convenient place to be anyway. We've been brought up to scorn campsites, to always go camping *au naturel*, 'wild camping' as it's now known. But the village site is fine. There are showers and loos and far fewer mosquitoes. We go to the little open-air ciné in the evening, sit on wooden benches in the hot moth-filled night. The movie is an ultra-violent spaghetti Western and we drink brandies afterwards at a bar strewn with peanut shells; I chew on a cheroot Clint Eastwood style and get Clare laughing.

It is in fact a great turning point for Spain, with Franco on his deathbed. For us on the ground, on the road, there's the lingering myth of the dangers of hitching in Spain with long hair and a rucksack – the danger all coming from the police side, Franco's fuzz, who bang up hippies and leave them to rot in jail. When I hitched down to Almeria with Lise in 1970 there seemed to be no such problem. We actually found it much easier to get rides than in France. The dangers were probably all there but we blithely ignored them.

Clare and I prefer to take trains in Spain, which are very cheap. We briefly mirror that other journey now: we look round Las Ramblas in Barcelona, take the overnight train to Valencia to save on accommodation, and next morning wander around the old part of the city. I may be hankering for my lost girl, but I'm also showing all these places I know to my sister on her first trip to Spain, first experience of independent foreign travel on a small budget. In lovely Valencia station, resting on the cool marble floor, we watch a gypsy family give a marvellous flamenco show – something I didn't see last time, despite it being one of our goals. So, one up for this trip. The passion of the music and dancing fill me with a wanderlust for the south again, but our money really is running low and we've college to get back to. So we turn inland, slowly cross the central plateau, taking local trains and hitching a little. We spend two days at the village of San Antonio by the railway track – a spaghetti Western kind of place – and do some art work. I still have my watercolour box and small block of paper in my backpack (it was my oil paints that were stolen in France). The dry land spotted with olive trees, the rows of vines marking out the hills, the deep blue sky, enrapture me as they always have. It seems to me my free on-the-spot watercolours aren't bad, like those done in the Scillies a few months before, but back at Falmouth, again no one else will think much of them. One problem, I learn, is my use of cold viridian for the olive trees. It's a difficult green and to be used with care. In my joy of the painting I've relaxed on colour, let my guard down – the free colour I use isn't quite the colour others see.

We hitch on across the burning plain. A Frenchman filled with some unknown venom for France and all things French tells us we must visit Toledo in preference to Madrid. An aristocratic Spaniard – immaculate suit and snow-white skin from *never* going out in the sun – drives us there. We walk across the bridge into the ancient hilltop town of Toledo without buying one of the innumerable paperknife swords on sale. We visit the dark churches, see the strange long-necked El Grecos, smell the cloying incense. Then, wandering narrow streets in the heat of afternoon, have our own experience of that place – a puppy stuffed into a plastic bag and left out to die in the sun. While hunting for pieces of painted pottery on some waste ground, we see the twitching carrier bag. I can only think of putting the wretched animal out of its misery. I pick up a rock, club its skull until it lies still. Weeping, we enter another hot, dark, incense-filled church with its gory, tortured Christ on the cross; a savage depiction of the crown of thorns, deep-gashed side, broken knees of the crucified.

We take a ferrobus to the edge of Madrid and sleep in an olive grove. Santa Cruz de la Zarza, by chance the very place I stopped with Lise – there are limited sleeping places available to the impecunious intent on sleeping rough outside the city. Next morning we wash in the restrooms of Madrid station and go to the Prado. On this second visit I'm most struck by Goya's *Black Paintings* of madness. I take another, better-informed look at Velasquez's *Las Meninas* with its tricks of mirrors and viewpoints, its puzzle of who's looking at whom. The picture is in such a fragile state now it can't be moved – you have to go there to see it. We believe we've found Picasso's *Guernica* too, but it proves to be a reproduction filling the space, waiting for the return of the original. Though Franco will die soon and *Guernica* be allowed back to Spain, The Museum of Modern Art in New York, custodian of the picture since the war, is keen to hang on to it and will drag out negotiations for several more years. The story of this bombed Basque town has an extra echo in our family as we are part Basque. Either a sixteeenth or a 'thirty-tooth', as we were told from a young age. This has always seemed special and exotic to me (and nothing to do with terrorism), though the information, which originally came from Granny Helen, has never been verified as far as I know.

Hitching on with Clare, north to Santander, following the 1970 route, I remember the randy Basque driver too – an unpleasant incident that happened late in the night when Lise and I were also on our way back. This square type in a white shirt with short back and sides hair, seemingly innocuous, picked us up after midnight, and started touching up Lise as she slept. Lise woke and yelled at him. We abandoned the car on a pitch-black road in the wilds of northern Spain. We blindly stuck out our thumbs at the next blazing headlights and got a lift to Santander.

This incident is strangely mirrored with Clare, and potentially much nastier. We have reached the north of Spain – Clare remembers a long coca-cola with lots of ice in Bilbao; I remember reaching the border at Iruna, flat broke. My notebook says we had only 27 pesetas left, such were the ridiculously small sums of money I managed to travel with then. We cross over into France and start hitching in the late afternoon. A lorry stops and offers us a ride all the way to Paris overnight. Great! A hitcher's dream. We settle down in the cab for the long night, Clare falling asleep in the driver's bunk. Then there's another lorry behind. Something starts up between the two drivers. They seem to be signalling to each other with their lights – those pre-mobile phone days. Our driver keeps looking in his wing mirror, dipping and undipping his headlights like some morse code. They're plotting something, they are after Clare, I'm suddenly sure of it. This time I'm more assertive. When our lorry pulls into an empty lay-by in the middle of nowhere and the lorry behind does the same, I spin into action, wake Clare, and without explanation bundle her out of the cab. We hurry away from the lights into the night and the lorries drive on –

they weren't stopping for a break. If we'd stayed in the cab, the other driver would have come round to the passenger door and got in. We stand huddled on the black road, the occasional car and lorry hurtling past, stick out our thumbs – and get our lift through to Paris.

19. The colour wheel

I start a painting of the harbour as soon as I get back. Ever since arriving in Falmouth I've been fascinated by the bay, its busyness and many boats; the giant tankers that come in to dock, so hugely out of scale with everything else; the elfin mirror dinghies that sail up against their hulks. It's an exhilarating, ever-changing variation of sky and light, wind and waves, rise and fall of tides.

The autumn weather is settled, water limpid and pearly bright. I start early in the morning, try to fix the picture's mood: a great black-hulled tanker tethered at dock, the yellow fields across the water at Flushing and further over the Carrick Roads to St Mawes looking unnaturally close. I take some photographs, make sketches and work in my room. It's still warm enough to swim. I run down to dip in the harbour below the house, dirty though it is, rather than trek out to the beach.

I'm still at Swanpool Street, and will be for all of my second year. Pasters is still in residence for the moment, which means his entourage too. The worldly American girlfriend has gone; his new friend hanging about is John Grimaldi from his St Albans school band Motiffe and now a virtuoso guitarist. Pasters is drummer in that band. Yorkshire Dave is around too, still wanting to show me his boat designs, and get in with Pasters. He follows them to the pub like a doleful spaniel. He's getting depressed in Falmouth. Some people sink here in Cornwall, however lovely it is. All too far away, isolating, and hostile to invading 'emmits' (anyone from across the Tamar). Dave is a melancholy sort anyway and the more he's excluded the worse he gets. While viewing the new boat plans in his attic, I look enviously at the rooftop views of the harbour. His room is full of light. I'm feeling stuck now in my back garden room among the yapping dogs.

When term begins I take the half-finished *Tanker* canvas up to the studios. I must try to settle there now. It's both my first painting away from the subject and first in the studios, a studio painting of course. My new space is a good size and overlooks the lawns and gardens, which I would also like to paint one day. There are screens on two sides from my neighbours, but I don't drape sheets over the entrance to hide myself from the corridor, no, I want people to come in.

And here's Dick Platt again, stammering some good news. I've won something. *Swanpool Street Interior* 3 has been commended for a Stowells Trophy.

Dick is so pleased. Falmouth has an unheard of four commendations this year. Star students Colin and Skeet, and a girl called Sylvie for her dark and romantic painting of horses. And me. It was Dick who put me in for the competition. It was the painter Carel Weight who picked me out during the summer term, when he came down to give a public crit on the best student work. We gathered in the hall with our paintings round the walls and Carel, shambling figure with a large rubbery face, prowled about making his comments. He praised my picture for its design, boldness, freshness, even for its colour.

My father also sends one of his minimal cards: 'I've been hearing good reports of your work down there.' Your father has only to say 'Quite good' occasionally for you to jump with joy. It can still happen when you're sixty.

My response to this success is to kill *Tanker*. Or so I'm told. Jumping ahead to Carel Weight's second crit, he singles out my canvas again – only to slam it. 'Now here's an example of an overworked picture. The colour in here is quite dead.' I'm shot through. I worked so long on this, worked hard at the colour. Have I painted it to death in the studio? Is it being away from the subject? Maybe I should always have the subject in front of me.

There's a colour course in November with Leo (Leo because she always wears a simulated leopardskin jacket). Suddenly anxious about it, whether even to do it, I tell Dick about my colour blindness at last, after a year at the college. He's surprised, he thinks I have rather a good sense of colour – I so want to believe him. No, I tell him, I can't actually see half the colours I put on the canvas. As Peter Cook might have put it: my optical cones are deficient in the red-green area. I'm *guessing*. It may be well-informed, but it's guesswork. The other staff haven't noticed either. But then no one ever said anything in all the time I was at Reading. Extraordinary, really. Ray is the only tutor I have told while out on our drawing trips – explaining why I work with charcoal all the time. Ray said I should just ignore it. Doesn't make any difference in the end. And looking at his work, the way he throws on the paint, I can see that it might not make much difference. Dick suggests I do a colour test up in the library.

So I take the Ishihara Test again, search for numbers concealed within circles of coloured spots. I first did this at school at the age of ten, when my colour blindness came to light in an art lesson – I'd painted the yeti from *Tintin in Tibet* green, thinking it was brown. The result is the same: red-green deficiency, indisputable. I talk to Leo. She says try the course anyway, some things will be useful if only in theory.

It's a relief to have come clean. My 'interesting' sense of colour has been getting a strain. Guesswork and luck, knowing how to mix a colour, looking at the label on the tube before squeezing it on the palette, trying to paint 'normally'. It's like painting by numbers, I almost laugh.

Colour blindness is inherited through the mother in missing

or damaged genes on the X chromosome. Females have two X chromosomes, males have an X and a Y – a missing stick from her second X chromosome becomes a Y, if you like. If a woman inherits a normal X as well as the mutated one, she won't show the mutation. Men, not having the second X to override the mutation, will. So colour blindness is much more common in men. The commonest kind, red-green, my kind, affects about 8% of men and .5% of women. My colour blindness comes through Mum then, as does my nephew's (Clare's son). We can't know if it came from her mother or her father, unless Teddy was colour-blind. If it was through Granny Betty it wouldn't show.

Dick looks at my Spanish watercolours. He notes the 'cold viridian'. I explain I was after the silvery grey-green of olive trees and making educated guesses at which colour to use, which is what I always do. Working in watercolour is all about colour and not much about tone, it highlights the problem. He points me to John Sell Cotman who painted his watercolours tonally and 'flat'. Then goes off and comes back with the name of a colour-blind Scottish artist he's unearthed (but only one).

Dad talks about tone. He says I'm a tonal painter and this is my strength – I probably see tone more accurately than most people. He cites Turner and Constable. Basically, the former is concerned with colour, the latter tone. I'd do better to look at Constable. I do look at Constable and love him, his 'willows, old rotten planks, slimy posts, and brickwork'. I've been to see his sketches in the V&A. In those greens and greys, the skies of fresh scudding clouds, there seems to me to be a love of nature as it really is. He speaks to me louder than the 'sublime' Turner. Though I do discover that there's a little question over Constable. It's an old chestnut and contentious. Did he add those obvious spots of red to the mass of greens because he was in fact colour blind? Cataracts seem more likely to me; the rather lurid quality of the greens in his late studio work might be down to the 'sheen of varnish' effect of having a cataract on his lens.

Hewlett says many painters use colour tonally – he does – and adds some French painters to the pot. Manet is tone and Renoir colour. Early Monets are tonal and late Monets colour, he says. Indeed, where the last great water lily paintings dissolve into a shimmer of pure colour is the point where my eyes let me down. And I do still long to 'see' Turner. I know I must be missing so much.

Dad again: 'No one knows how others see colour. We all see colours differently. It's possible you see some colours more accurately than people with normal vision.'

But I don't want these allowances. I have to admit that the vivid green stripe on my commended Stowell's painting, which may work well, may even clinch the picture in Carel Weight's view, was not me being 'bold and daring' in colour. It was a happy accident. It may have been bold in design but colourwise I was just trying to make a shadow by mixing blue into the yellow ochre I'd used for the wood. Sometimes it works, sometimes it doesn't – as with everyone, surely, from Picasso down. The difference with me though, is in being unable to *know* whether the colour works or not.

Nevertheless I approach Leo's course with great seriousness and hope, really. I study the colour wheel: complementary, secondary and tertiary colours; warm and cool colours, saturation and tint. I learn that jumping across the wheel between complementaries will produce vibrancy and zing, whereas moving to adjacent colours will be quiet, harmonious. I learn you get black by mixing the three primary pigments (and white by mixing the light primaries), and how difficult it is to make a pure black in paint. Terry Frost talked about it in Reading; he doesn't use black from the tube, he mixes his own blacks. I of course can't do that. It impinges directly on the problem. I don't know whether my mix is a green-black, red-black or purple-black.

I'm interested in how the complementaries zing against each other. I get it clearly with blue and orange, my strong colours, but less so with the others. Red-green retains its mystery for me – those holly berries that vanish against the same tone green of the leaf. With purple-yellow I see the blue of the purple and the orange of the yellow, I shift round the circle. I do this with reds and greens to some extent – the green towards blue, the red towards orange – and get some zing. It's less than for those with standard colour vision but nonetheless still exciting. So in *Tanker* I kept adding touches of orange to the blue of the water, building up these resonant greys. I kept the tones very close to accentuate the small differences. Then I lost it, couldn't see it, or not all of it. Other things were happening, I was told, beyond my range of vision. Some nice touches of pink had appeared in the water, for example. *What pink?* This actually has much to do with the properties of the pigments themselves, the tubes of colour, which don't perfectly fit the colour wheel. The blue and orange I used mixed to a *pinkish* grey (apparently) but then it was gone. I'd obliterated the delicate pink without even seeing it.

If there's a fault now, it's in my not coming fully clean with myself. I still try not to let my handicap spoil the painting. I want to keep that pink even if I can't quite see it – because someone has liked it, has praised it. This is like refusing to 'murder your darlings' when writing a poem; the good bit, the bit you're so proud of, is the bit that has to go. It's actually holding you back, this precious bit, getting in the way and stopping you move on. But I'm kidding myself about seeing the colour I 'know' I've mixed – like searching for the number concealed among the Ishihara spots and imagining it. There's a lot of mind work going on in visual perception. Like the reversed image of a face in a mould or inside a mask which appears positive because you know faces so well. We do indeed tend to see what we want to see.

So I work with labels and knowledge to try to overcome the problem. In my notebooks I calculate how to use colour, get effects with colour, how to mix colours. Greens are my bugbear. There are lists for mixing all colours but especially greens. Monestial or Prussian Blue + a yellow = Chrome Green, + Cobalt Yellow = Hooker's Green, + Raw Sienna = a sap green; + Burnt Sienna for deep olive, for toning down a yellow; Viridian, a brilliant transparent green in thin layers, a blackish body colour in impasto. It's funny to see these lists now, a bit sad too.

Of course I see colour, but I see *my version*, as my father said. And it *is* interesting that no one really knows what colour another sees. We approximate, imagine and *think* colours all the time. And I'm learning about these colours I see or don't see. I prefer Braque's soft palette, say, to Matisse's sumptuous one, or Picasso's harsh one. And though I must be missing much in a Rothko painting, perhaps I do see more of the texture, the soft feather edges, the generous brushstrokes in compensation.

I appreciate the good colourists around me – Kate, Simon, John Magoldrick. I seem to be able to pick a painting which has good colour without being able to name its colours. I appreciate the tones and add a bit of colour theory. I might know too much colour theory. What I long for is the real thing, the feeling of colour, which these colourists have. I don't have it and I can't buy it.

One thing I could do is really 'throw the paint'. I could hurl colours at the canvas and to hell with the result. Work in random mad colour! I will do something like this in my next painting, *Black Range*, but not enough, and it haunts me. For surely that's what Kate did when she gave up painting. She shouted at it, sent it packing, and moved on. I will have another go at throwing the paint in a few years' time.

I go for a tea in the canteen. The queue stretches round two walls and inching my way round towards the counter is ten minutes of drastically slowed time. Suddenly I don't know where to *be.* Which table shall I sit at? There are no tables I can comfortably join at all. *Look, you've just come up from the studio for a cup of tea, why don't you take it back there?* I carry my tea to the safety of my space.

I stop at the shop to get more white paint.

'Bit of Tit White for you, John?' chirps John from Dartmouth.

No, Flake,' I counter and he winces, swallowing the poison like Van Gogh. Flake White of course contains lead – remember the weight of the tube? – and it comes with health warnings now. Dirty John's Titanium has taken over from Flake. I don't smile at his daily tit joke as I could. I just cringe and feel the old grimace back on my face.

It's happening again. There has been a downward turn ever since getting back from Spain, hasn't there, and I don't know why, there's no apparent reason … Is it too much time spent painting? Am I just a depressed character like Dave the boat builder? No, I'm not! Nothing has actually happened, I tell myself over and over, but I feel myself sinking. Fog creeping into the harbour. The world closing in on me again. The last time was the summer I arrived in Falmouth fifteen months ago. A recurrence of that then, is it? I fear it.

Oh I fear being like my mother who gets a severe depression most years. It's hardly in the notebooks, just discernable between the lines, but she was in Tone Vale this summer for four weeks, and will be again next summer for a massive nine weeks. She has shock treatment both times. I don't want that.

20. A gap in the hedge

Lionel Miskin, Complementary Studies tutor, is approaching, tall and willowy down the hill. He's wearing a richly-toned, probably green suit today. I have a moment of panic, long to run through the gap in the hedge just there. It's the shortcut home, through into a cul-de-sac and up to the main road; I use it when I can't face meeting all the college people on the hill. Today I have a line from *Prufrock* ready in my head to prepare a face to meet the faces that you meet, and hold my ground. What on earth's the point in running away from Lionel? He's the one offering to help me through these freak-outs.

When he sees me he seems to hesitate too. His long body appears to lean away, his head inclines at an angle like a heron. He slows but doesn't stop, murmurs, 'Things okay?' and carries on down the hill. They aren't really, no. I turn and hurry after him.

I catch him at the noticeboard, stroking his moustache. Stand beside the dark knobbly jacket. 'D'you like it?' he says. 'They give me such stick about this suit. Spinach they call it! How *are* you?'

I don't like the way he announces me at the busy noticeboard and quietly ask if it's okay to come and see him. I've been offered 'a chat about things' with Lionel, whose other role at the college is pastoral care. He nods. 'How about Wednesday afternoon?'

'We've got some rather good movies this term,' he goes on, examining the film list. 'And by the way, I can recommend Peter Redgrove's talk coming up. The Wise Wound. Fascinating.'

The foyer is suddenly swarming and Lionel is carried away towards the canteen in a stream of women, it seems to me. I walk back up the hill, not through the gap in the hedge today, but still back to my room. Why aren't I going into the canteen for a coffee and Danish pastry with all these women?

The fog rolls in. I begin to fear going out again. Even leaving my room. I emerge for essentials only and then scurry back in. I don't go to a doctor this time. I tell my family by letter – Frank and Clare, and I suppose my father. I must have written to him saying I was feeling 'a bit deppy' because he replies with some sympathy, saying many students have 'difficulties' in their second year but generally they get over them. It helps a little – and I am glad for the recognition that this mood might not be entirely of my own making – but it hardly makes a difference.

I go to see Lionel at the end of October. After our first talk I write:

Go slowly. Ease your way through, don't fight struggle. Relax, give yourself time. Gently prod into your family where all the problems spring from. Inferiority is the lion and the mouse. Don't try to be the lion. A balance between the two. Masturbate if you are hungry without guilt. Record your dreams. The Greek myth of a four-armed monster split into two by the gods, which spends its time trying to get back together into oneness, is about sexuality.

A letter arrives from Frank the following week.

Dear John
Have just got your letter and as I'm early this morning here is a quick reply. We are terribly sorry to hear 'Black Dog' – as Churchill called it – has descended again. I'm sure there is nothing to do but what you are doing – retreat into your stronghold and wait for it to go again. It will, probably sooner than you think. We would <u>much</u> rather you wrote than kept quiet about it. In some ways the more people you confide in the better. I think it would help to see a doctor. You don't have

to take his pills, though in a bad patch it might be a good thing to do.

I keep changing my attitude to pills. Obviously we mustn't all become dependent on them but these black passages are chemical, some minute change or build up in the nervous system, and so it is not unreasonable to take something to correct the balance. Gradually more will be known about the chemistry, and the cure will be more certain. Why not ask to see a psychiatrist? They know what is available.

We are coping here. I think Mum's injection is helping but it is too early to say. Not drinking and losing weight anyway!

Sarah's birthday is on 16th. A card would go down well.

Granny's tax problems at last sorted out. She only owes them £52. She had feared thousands. New worry is her eyes.

Must go. Don't think about your depression or try to reason it out. It gets nowhere. Get by from day to day.

All good wishes, Frank.

I sit in my room with the letter. Through the window Mrs Birch is contemplating her eucalyptus trees. She still has four. In the summer she was mourning the loss of the largest one, blown down in a gale, but we uprighted it with ropes and now it's sprouting again. The two saplings in the middle of the garden have doubled in size in a year. And the neighbours *have* voiced worries about their view of the harbour being blocked, but she ignores them. Frank is a marvel. Even if he has moved out of their bedroom and into mine – to get away from Mum/get a better night's sleep. I am indeed lucky to get such a letter. I sit on my arse with his letter in my hand, staring out of the window, and time ticks by.

I see a student counsellor rather than a psychiatrist. We meet in an elegant room in Rosehill overlooking the college gardens, sit opposite each other at a small table by the window. After introductions, we grind to a silence. The man is waiting for me to speak. This is Cognitive Therapy. It has to come from me. But I don't/can't/won't say anything. The strange, pregnant silence (for which he is getting paid) goes on and on. I suppose I must have given in and spoken in the end, but he doesn't give me anything useful in return. I just resent his trying to make me break and blurt out, for extracting things from me in such a soulless way.

I have another of these sessions, then decide to stick with Lionel and Jung. I'm sceptical about Jung (and remain so to this day – maybe Freud gets closer by simply reducing everything down to sex). But I do want to talk more with Lionel, so will suffer the Archetypes for him.

Lionel is fascinating, intense, birdlike; a heron or egret, or snake-eating secretary bird of South Africa in a spinach-green suit. I look around his wonderful room, a true cornucopia of objects; many ceramics and figurines; any number of books on art and film.

He introduces me to the Spoiler, the Topdog, the Internal Saboteur – he has several names for this little devil: the one who always tries to stop you. The one who doesn't want you to do any painting (let alone win a prize), who doesn't want you to even get out of bed. He's someone who must be dealt with, and he's right inside you.

'Dreams are the key,' says Lionel, 'and I'd very much like to hear some of yours.'

Fancy someone caring enough to look at my dreams. Lionel wants me to 'catch' as many as I can and suggests a little 'strategy': drink a glass of water before bed and have a notebook ready for when I wake up for the loo, hopefully in mid-dream.

This works. I do catch many dreams, many bits and fragments of dreams. I even get into the groove, as Lionel hoped, of being 'ready' while still in my dream to jot it down.

I will continue with this dream-catching for years. Dispense with the pint of water but keep a notebook to hand by the bed. It's likely that my morning diary habit, kept daily for most of the last twenty-five years, came out of this. I like to write it first thing, often bleary with sleep. It's a kind of writer's diary, a tool, a way into my subconscious as I wake fresh from dreams before any censors come down.

You write your feelings and moods when you're young and blue, as my mother puts it. I don't need any encouragement from Lionel to do this. As a child I kept sporadic but quite detailed diaries of holidays with my father. I've kept up regular nature notes at Colham. Now, out it all flows. In amongst the purple sandpipers and black redstarts go pieces of my own natural history. What I don't do is put a date to them, or even bother to put them in order. I just open the book on a clean page and scribble. So the words are all over the place, difficult to place.

I bring Lionel my bits and pieces of dreams.

> A French stick spotted with mould. A battered top hat in the corner of a cupboard. An owl flew up from under my feet.

> Painting in a field near Redruth, a girl came up and asked for my autograph (she recognised me from my exhibition). I signed my name very small in a corner of the page, unlike all the other exuberant signatures.

> My only exhibit in the show was a small pencil drawing of the back of my head.

> In the workshop with Dartmouth John. I was mending an enormous white wardrobe … suddenly I was interested in making a sculpture out of pins and paper of an 'Impressionist

lady' in a flounced dress. I worked quickly and surely, knew it was right. John laughed at my sculpture, so ridiculously small compared to the wardrobe.

Lionel suggests the white wardrobe is my mother and I'm astonished. Am I trying to mend her? Could be.

Tim Holiday says dreams are just the things we can't make sense of during the day.

Lionel says the purpose of dream analysis is for the unexpected associations they throw up which couldn't come from the conscious. There's no magic in them. He knows I'm suspicious of magic.

In a pub for ages not knowing anyone. Somebody said 'Smell this' and put a brandy under my nose. It was Kate. I inhaled the brandy fumes, felt them surge through me. I asked how she could afford brandies in a pub, she said she saved up and made a night of it. She produced a pound and told me to buy more and some 'brandy crispies'. I went to the bar, got two brandies, started drinking mine – it was delicious, strong. But I'd forgotten the crispies. At last I got the barman's attention but I'd gone blank, couldn't remember what I wanted. At last I remembered and alone now returned with the drinks, and fell flat on the floor. My friend Mark Fry was beside me with a basket. He helped me up and we put the crispies in the basket and they turned into cardboard soldiers he'd just bought at a jumble sale. Then the pub was taken over by college people and I couldn't get back to Kate.

Crazy dreams, what are they? But Lionel listens and there's value in that. It's good just to look at them in daylight, reconstruct the images. I must look at painters who have painted their dreams. Artists like Chagall are a lot more understandable when you see them from a dream perspective. Look at Surrealism.

Lionel runs a film night as part of his Complementary Studies and if my dreams run dry he's always ready to talk about cinema from Bunuel to Dalí to Tarkovsky. He will show me *The Discreet Charm of the Bourgeoisie* – Bunuel's surreal fun-poking at middle-class mores is pure Lionel. He'll shock me with the excruciating razor scene in *Un Chien Andalou.* Intrigue and entice me with *The Mysteries of the Organism.* Liberate me with his friend Lindsay Anderson's vitriolic attack on public schools in the film *If.* Empathise with me over the horror version of mental health care that is *One Flew Over the Cuckoo's Nest*, while Mum goes in and out of mental hospital.

And Lionel's running a yoga class this term. I go along – maybe we all try yoga as students. I've had a go before and didn't get far. 'Try again. Fail again. Fail better,' as Beckett said. Lionel is also valiantly taking part. I watch him battle with his 'stiff English legs' that are just like mine, skinny, knobbly-kneed, and refusing to comply with the mind's vision of them as supple things that will bend and flex and soon slip into the lotus position; indeed they find it hard enough to stay crossed for more than a few minutes. The yoga business is as painful and unproductive as ever for me. Lying on my back to relax, settling my breathing before a meditation exercise, I fall asleep. At least I'm relaxed. I manage a couple more sessions, practise hard for a while, and gain a little ground. I more or less achieve a half-lotus position but never a full one with both knees on the floor, and let it peter out.

I go back to my room and do a fourth Swanpool Street interior, my black throw-the-paint interpretation of the old iron cooking range built into the wall. I mix my own blacks, stir everything into the mix. *Black Range* is another Braque-influenced work on sand. Coming through Paris with Clare in the summer, I saw some of my favourite Braques in the flesh: the *Billiard Tables*, the *Studio* series. How they leapt out at you, physical, tangible, objects in themselves. Now I pile on the paint, mix more sand into the paint, build it up over several weeks. It becomes very thick and … black.

I abandon the thing in the end. It has just become a vehicle for my doom and gloom, a surface to chuck things at, and I don't think much of it at all. So what a surprise and honour, when I leave Falmouth, that Dick should ask if they could have *Black Range* for the staff room. I wonder how long it stayed up.

Clare writes, thanking me for my 'honest letter', in full sympathy for my Black Dog, and with much of her own to say. Her life is suddenly full. She's in love. She tells me what she held back during our Spanish journey.

> I'm sitting in the Slade in front of two of my pictures trying to decide whether they are finished! They're the strongest I've ever done – bright, lush, thick; red, blue, yellow, black, chocolate brown and white. Verticals and diagonals for the first time on a large scale. Some canvas collage, hard and soft edges. Very physical. I feel so much more now … since the end of last summer (when I reached as near the edge as I've ever been – Catherine rescued me) I've not been on my own. First Catherine came to live with me, then you on holiday, and since then Richard and I have been together. He is warm and gentle and always smiling (even if sometimes as a nervous reaction). Things go from there. I'm living a lot more in the same amount of time, in fact all the time! I've spread myself to the edges …
>
> Of course we should go home for Christmas. That for Mum would be a final abandonment. Frank has left her in a way by moving into your room to sleep. Catherine rang me up last weekend, a great and welcome surprise. She seemed well but lonely. It was hard to tell her about Richard. He was her dream romance. It was all so strange and Freudian, her, Richard and

I in London that week before you came, after a very eventful party … She has been home and had to leave as she felt she was cracking up. Apparently Mum is having even more pills and drinking again, which Frank has now discovered. I've given up, I try hard not to think about it, though often I can't help it. I'm like her in the way I'm subject to outside conditions. Though I'm more in control of those conditions, which I think is the key. Mum is totally dependent on other people, Frank really. She really never has been herself. No one has ever given her a chance. I don't think she could take it now even if it was offered. That sounds terrible – no one should ever be that isolated.

Ray comes round in late November. He's choosing a picture from his lock-up to put in for the Royal Academy's next summer show.

'God, you look rough,' he says. 'Are you okay?'

I tell him I am, it's nothing. We get some of the enormously heavy paintings out and prop them around the yard. He makes his choice – a tumultuous Kokoschkan landscape with giddy skies – and prices it up by size and weight, according to his system. It comes to several hundred pounds.

'Not so expensive,' he objects. 'You have to take into account all the time spent doing the ones which don't get exhibited. They all lead up to this moment.'

He doesn't get his picture in this year. Sometimes he does, he strikes lucky. It's all a lottery. Art's a rum business, he says, as Turner once said while actually in the Academy adding finishing touches to his work even as his show opened. I wonder how Ray got his painting up to Piccadilly. Did he strap it to the roof of his van? Take it by train to Paddington in the guard's van and then taxi? Then, unsold, all the way back to his lock-up.

I will be delivering two of Frank's paintings to the RA. I

have them ready with me. The very opposite of a Ray Atkins. Miniatures. Tiny geometric patterns, amazingly detailed and intricate, repeated round a square at the centre, radiating out. Like a fine Persian carpet, like a mandala. More than a hundred hours for each one, I'd say, with a fine sable brush. And he gets both paintings in. He sells them. He's enormously pleased, especially when one of the buyers writes to express her joy in his 'jewel-like' work. Makes it all worthwhile, he smiles, all those hours spent at the tempestuous kitchen table. Frank, so self-deprecating about his amateur little paintings, is given this fresh beacon of hope.

Just before Christmas I'm in London again, staying with Clare, with Clare and Richard. I've run there from Falmouth according to my diary, but the trip was at least partly planned because it includes my delivery to the Royal Academy. I just hand them over in the basement, where all the entries are arriving by car and van and taxi, these small precious offerings of Frank's, and they vanish into strange hands. I go on to *New Work* 2 at the Hayward Gallery. I like the 'Brutalist' rough concrete textures of the Hayward. It's one of those mixed shows with a bit of everything, like a degree show, but I enjoy some white plaster and wood sculptures by Peter Startup, and look at Constructivist artist Malcolm Hughes because Clare knows him at the Slade. The work is more modern than Falmouth, closer to Reading. I visit Housmans Bookshop on the Caledonian Road and buy *The Ecologist* magazine's *A Blueprint for Survival* and *The Environmental Handbook: Action Guide for the UK* published by the embryonic Friends of the Earth: 'Your last chance to make Britain worth living in'. I've given up my degree with the OU, but still follow the new ecology movement.

At Clare's I dream of a family holiday with Dad and Catherine H in a village by a river in Cornwall. They had two young children now. Dad was very jolly, livening us up, bringing us together, but this new family didn't work. Then I dream of a grand journey with my old girlfriend to Spain. On a long straight dusty road, we were making love, high, in continuous orgasm; detouring to Bulgaria to meet a friend, Johnnie. Two girlfriends of his arrived and we were all swept up into ecstasy again.

There was much more. I only ever seem to catch smallest parts of dreams; the great epic thing swirls away out of reach. I don't believe that the bit you remember is necessarily the most important; it's just the point at which you happen to wake up and so retain – when the dog barks, the doorbell rings, a foghorn sounds in the bay. I wake in a sweat with one of my toes bleeding from thrashing around in the bed from reliving (or relieving) the Spanish journey with Lise. It was a dream I didn't want to wake up from.

I visit her and De Gruyter when I'm in London. They have their own small house together now, something I won't embark on for another eight years. They are settled, and this is somehow confirmed by playing tennis with them on the hard court at the end of their garden – the court doesn't belong to them, we crawled through the hedge and wire netting. I'm pleased that they have my *White Rectangle with Apple* sculpture from Reading on the piano. My sister Catherine has also visited. She's been in contact with Lise for a while, seeking advice, someone to talk to. Lise sees trouble ahead if Catherine continues to live at home. She really has to get herself out of there. Lise is full of sympathy but, in the end, sighs, she can only do so much.

It's true what Lise said – we're too close and involved with my sister to be able to help properly. She needs new blood from outside, a strong consistent dose of normal life which forces her to live, to choose and be responsible for herself. Mum never grew up emotionally and somehow all the 'help' – the years of treatment and drugs – has stopped her ever leaving her childhood; now she's only half alive, her real self buried so far down it seems she'll never come up again. Catherine mustn't be allowed to go down that same road.

I go to the Slade Christmas party with Clare and Richard.

'Ladies ...' crows the master of ceremonies in his coat and tails. 'Ladies, ladies, ladies. Welcome, my charming, lovely, beau-ti-ful ladies. Ladies and ladies ...' Hilariously he goes on without ever reaching any gentlemen. I don't know what to do at this party. I wander off with my drink down the corridors filled with sculpture busts and figures, 'the antique'. I think of Mum at the Slade, when she was happy, she said. A right party girl in those days by her own admission. In the album at home there's a photo of her from 1947 resplendent in a ball gown on the steps outside. It was just before she met Dad.

He was here too, walking these same corridors. They put him in the corridor, he said, because he was 'abstract' and the rooms were all given over to life painting. But he worked from the model too, as you had to then. He described 'eccentric' Lucian Freud, who came to teach once a week, entering the life room where everyone was clustered round the model. Freud crept around, back against the wall, sometimes came forward to whisper something in a student's ear – the sum of his teaching back in 1950, as Dad remembers. 'And he was well paid for it!' As it turned out my father would go on to share his first exhibition with Lucian Freud. It was Freud and Froy at the Hanover Gallery in 1951, one upstairs, one down.

I don't know where I spent Christmas Day. I hope it was at Waterloo Road together with my sisters for Mum's sake. As Clare said in her letter, we mustn't abandon her. On Boxing Day at least I'm back home and calling it 'a resting place, a lull between real places, warm and cosy'. I only outwardly prefer

Colham, I think. I really want the warmth of my mother's home with its Frank protection.

One of my New Year's resolutions is to give up the guitar: 'this mechanical plodding.' My affair with the classical guitar goes back to leaving school and beginning with Lise, and I see now this decision was some kind of final severing. So, a positive move. But I would be losing out on playing at Colham and with Vic at Falmouth. The peak of my classical guitar work was our William Lawes duet, which we never quite finished before he left last year.

I also resolve to jump in at the deep end to deal with my depression. To use more of Lionel's 'strategies and games' to find ways round problems. I must keep my place on the ladder. I've become very aware of this business with the ladder: the more you step down, the harder it is to step back up.

21. Big black cloud

A month later I'm back at Waterloo Road, this time on the way to collect my Stowell's award. I will be staying with Clare in London as usual. I asked Lise and De Gruyter to put me up again and this time was refused. Maybe they are busy this weekend, maybe not, but I can quite see why I shouldn't go back there so soon. But should I be going to London at all? Why not skip it and just stay here? Who wants this poxy award anyway? The Spoiler is active: he doesn't want me to receive my prize. No, yes, no. Go … home. Suddenly I wanted to be at home again.

I arrange a lift with a guy called Yves – so whatever the doom and gloom in my diary, I'm still functioning reasonably well. Yves drops me at the Wellington bypass and I give him a pound for petrol. I walk home the back way across the fields, pass the chrysanthemum nursery where I had a summer job. Those weird irradiated colours they were getting by 'nuking' the plants at Hinkley Point are like the weird colours in my paintings now. I shut the Spoiler up and see a potential painting in the two oaks by the gate, the way they stand sentinel against the western skyline.

My arrival surprises Frank and Sarah, both for its lateness and unexpectedness. I didn't warn them – I don't. Waterloo Road is my 'open house' where I can turn up whenever I want, something I can't do at my father's.

But Catherine is calling me from upstairs, urgently. She stays on the stairs and I stay talking to Frank in the hall, unable to register that my sister needs me. It's me, surely, who needs help now. It's our mother who needs help – Mum isn't well at the moment, she's up in bed, and that's no surprise. Suddenly Catherine is sobbing in my arms. We stand there hugging in the hall, something we've hardly done before, and it's a hugging we both need. We go into the kitchen, sit and talk about what's wrong. We have symptoms in common: indecision, fixations – unreasonable clinging to an idea. We're scared of things, everything. We sleep a lot, can't get up in the morning.

After twenty-four hours the balance has tilted. My sister is doing all the leaning and I'm doing the listening. She's possessive of my time, wants every minute of it. I feel I'm deserting her by going off to play a game of chess with Frank. This is draining me. I grow impatient and stop listening to her. I feel it's contagious too, that her troubles are piling on top of my own.

I go next door to phone Clare. Granny's in a perky mood. 'I've finished *War and Peace*! Going to read it again now.'

She doesn't get on my nerves like Mum. I don't mind her pottiness. Maybe it's because I'm always a visitor now and don't have to put up with the daily grind; there isn't time to irritate each other. Granny's rereading of *War and Peace* has become our little joke.

'Having a good rest?'

She eyes me, knows I'm not. I feel exhausted at home, not rested. She tells me not to set my sights too high, not all at once. She's astute, Granny. I want to talk about me, cry, but I can't do that with her. She'd have no truck with that. I can't cry with anyone here. I can't with my sister Catherine after all, nor with young Sarah – so young for all this. And never really with my stepfather, Frank. The only one I could cry with is with my mother, the shadowy figure upstairs.

I watch a *World About Us* documentary on the peregrine falcon. Apart from the bird being so beautiful, so perfectly made to fit its niche, the people in the film are also doing something real and meaningful. I want to be a social worker for birds not humans.

I have a dream which I could record but feel myself refusing.

I won't make the effort to turn on the light and pick up a pencil. It was long and complex and I know has plenty in it, but that's *all* I can remember. Of course it fades away like smoke.

My job on Monday is to escort Catherine into her A-level exam. This has been arranged in advance. She asked me to take her to the Tech, to physically get her there, because she wouldn't be able to make herself. In the end I almost had to force her. We're in the County Stores in Taunton after lunch, twenty minutes before the start of the exam, and suddenly she announces she isn't going to do the exam. By five to two I have cajoled and persuaded her. We set off running to the Tech at the edge of town and someone is there to lead her into the examination room ten minutes late. I remember her face paralysed with fear.

I go on to London and straight through the Stowell's ceremony in a daze. Collect my medal, and get back to Clare and Richard's. That same evening there's a phone call from Doctor Richardson – about Catherine. He has never called Clare in London before; he's actually at Granny's with Catherine. She froze up in the exam, sat there for an hour and wrote nothing, poor girl. Now she's going to collapse in bed, no doubt under sedation, until Clare arrives on Thursday night.

When I get back to Cornwall, it's all still there of course. Everything I ran away from falls right back on top of me. I have a fresh supply of pills from Richardson but am resistant to taking them. I can't be like Mum. She takes so many of these pills.

I do some yoga, meditating if you like, on Saturday afternoon.

Sit still with eyes closed. A stream of images, ideas, possibilities appear and disappear. Some are important, some not. I can hardly distinguish between them. They all have equal value to me, these fleeting thoughts that come and go. I know I must get myself out of this state but am unable to grasp any single idea before getting swamped in all the rest … Indecision has been bad today. The effort to make a decision insurmountable. I can get over one or two obstacles, but there are always more, and they are stronger in the end. So I don't do anything.

Must must get up early and work a full morning in the college, five days.

On Monday morning I walk up to college to sign in. What a fiasco that turns into. This is Black Dog, full-on. Back in my room I write down the experience. I'm trying to describe it for someone, for Lionel. Last year I wrote about A Day in the Life of My Mother, now I write one about myself.

> First feelings were good, cleaned out, as they often are after plenty to drink the night before. Breakfast was okay, I was grateful to think about the basics, what to stuff in my gob. Before going out I double-checked I had everything, esp. pipe, tobacco and matches, and managed to make myself a bit late as usual, so I'd meet fewer people on the way into college.
>
> I passed B on the other side of the road and successfully avoided him – the bend in the road meant I could look straight ahead and not 'see' him. R was unavoidable, especially as we'd sat at the same table in the pub last night (though didn't speak). Managed a fairly bright 'Morning' to him. Then Lionel drove past, daydreaming in his camper van. Could have asked him about the bird man he told me about; he's trying to help me.
>
> Ducked into college to sign in. Leafy and Judy were just going in and I had to greet them. *I used to know them.* They're both in Pasters' band now, and Judy gave me an encouraging smile. I like her Texan drawl and the denim boiler suits she wears, though not her hairy legs. She deliberately doesn't shave them. I rushed ahead up the stairs as if in a hurry, as if very busy. In the office I kept my back turned to them, hunted in my pocket for things, and left.

Now worked up into my usual state, a kind of whirlwind of fear, I headed away from the college to the town library. C and D passed me – another of my ghastly smiles was met with a hard stare from C (good for him, not scared off). I accelerated away down the street, head down, eyes on feet, to get past people quicker.

At the top of Jacob's Ladder I remembered a year-old idea for a painting. Saw it again, more clearly: the ivy leaves in close-up on the surface of the picture plane, the long flight of steps in exaggerated perspective. I'd do it, really try. I watched the will to do it dissolve away even as I went down the steps. No, don't want to do that. Can't. Too hard. Oh depression is a lazy thing. I know it's lazy even though I'm inside it. It's like helplessly knowing you're in a dream. You're giving up painting, aren't you? Then you won't have to do all this mental work. There, end of problem.

I still hadn't reached the library. Had to make a detour to the post office for stamps. Question: should I queue at the post office? To queue or not to queue. Yes, queue, get the fucking stamps. I want to write to people.

The library at last. Bird books. Something on hides so I can photograph birds close up. Build a hide of canvas and wood, camouflage it, take it right down to the water's edge.

I was a long time looking, picking up books on other subjects. A boy came in and checked through the bird books, found nothing he wanted and left. Simple. I went into the reference library. More time passed, safely, in a dream. Couldn't take out any of these anyway. I finally chose two books. Then, absurd moments, I'd lost my library card. Fumbling, apologies, dropped letters and stamps, a £5 note blowing about on the floor, before I found it.

On my way back to my room. I was going to Tesco's for something. Too late, past it now. The baker's? Yes. Optician's?

> No. Bookshop? It was empty and the girl watched me as I passed. No. Greengrocer's? Don't know. Home at last. Noon already. I gave in and took a Valium, first of the day, the absolute wreck of the day so far. The drug takes hold, slows me down, makes me sleepy. Things are neither good nor bad. No, they are better.

I have to think about my Complementary Studies project, which isn't run by Lionel but by Tim. You can do anything you like for this. There seems to be total freedom of subject matter. I hate this freedom, can't possibly take advantage of it at the moment. I want parameters, to be told what to do. OK then, I'll design a house, my perfect house ... I sketch a fantasy house built into a hillside, melding in with the slope, with minimum disturbance to nature. Actually, it's a progression from my teenage 'hobbit hole' with round green front door and shiny brass knocker. But modern, with clean lines of glass and wood, a plain rectangle from the front, a triangle from the side. There's no garden or fence – nature is the garden. In the Blueprint for Survival we must go with nature not against it. I site my new eco house at the head the rabbit valley at Colham. That's to say, just outside my father's valley.

Lionel cracks the knuckles of his long fingers. 'Any more dreams?'

I had a party dream – I often have party dreams. I think: my mother loves parties and I criticise her shallowness, yet I dream about parties. I've had a whole *series* about parties with my childhood friend Mark, through which I gradually move from feeling the outsider to being accepted. In one dream I have a girlfriend at last and can now take on various opponents, outdo them in guitar playing and sword fighting. They try to belittle me, make me 'little old John' again, but by the end I know I'll win. Mark has made a tape of my guitar performance and plays it to the audience, now standing in a wood.

And there's a Colham dream:

> Carol, Sarinda, Lizzie, Diane arrived from Falmouth one by one. We watched the TV which was now on the other side of the fireplace. Dad's log fire was blazing but everyone turned away from it. Embarrassment all round. I felt responsible but couldn't act. Dad was out in the kitchen, cooking. I kept thinking he would intervene, come and be the lively host. Then we left in a minibus, Dad driving. After a long drive uphill we came to a junction with a vast traffic jam, noise and hooting like on the way to Padstow. We learnt we were on our way to New York.

I've been to the May Day celebrations over in Padstow – a long day in and out of the pubs (open all day), much of it with Simon, following the swirling black 'Obby 'Oss through the narrow streets of the own. The beat of drums, the endless round of the May Day song – 'for summer is acome unto day': never forgotten – ringing through our drunken heads. Simon went off with his dancing girlfriend, I think, and I ended the day alone … Four Falmouth women in one dream, I could talk about them.

'You really want to hear all these dreams, Lionel?'

'Do you really want to tell me?'

We've been doing dreams for a while now, and I'm not sure where it's going. It seems to me Lionel adds meanings of his own, or of Jung's. He says the big white wardrobe I dreamt about is my mother, but I don't know whether it is or not. Why can't it just be a wardrobe? I'm inclined to say, facetiously, that of course you can say my mum, any mother, is some kind of container or receptacle. Maybe she's the bottle of brandy she swigged and hid behind the dustbin. And my dad. How is 'a glacier in the Japanese style'?

‘Yes, do go on.’ His eyes are closed. ‘I’d like you to tell me. Jung tells us the way to get over these inner conflicts of ours is not to fight with them, but get above them and reconcile the opposites.’

> I was on the way from home to Clare’s new flat. Down a country lane, past a house full of furniture – all empty drawers, I checked. I wanted to stay behind, look longer, but we hurried on to her place. It was palatial, we went up past a luxurious first floor to a second with an enormous noisy wooden hall and clattery stairs – not hers but for returned servicemen, with the smell of stale tobacco like a barber’s – and upstairs again to her flat …
>
> Earlier. Charlotte, holding her tiny beautiful hand and wrist. We had sex. We set off for Italy on a boat.

It’s about empty Colham, isn’t it? and Clare’s large London flat with its bare wooden stairs, and me getting off with Charlotte after all, unlike in real life, and seeming to want to return to Italy. Is it about anything else? He seems to be asleep.

‘I dreamt I was working in a huge factory, Lionel, moving objects from place to place. I saw Edmund Boulting, no, his twin Rupert, and remembered him from school. He looked through me. I feigned surprise and greeted him heartily, overacting – he was a leader, strong, active, handsome, and I always envied him. It was Rupert I got on with, more than his brother. But he didn’t reply to my greeting, he continued to ignore me, slowly got on with his job. He looked sad, lost, pathetic, but somehow beautiful and noble too. I suddenly knew he was on heroin. I tried to see his arms but they were tightly buttoned at the wrist. I held his wrists but couldn’t look for the needle marks. He was so beautiful and fragile and precious.’

This is a hangover dream, the morning after a party. We

talked about drugs at the party. The wrists were about when a policeman once stopped and searched me for drugs in London. I admired Rupert at school when I was eleven, twelve. I tried harder to be his friend than he did me – he had so many friends. He once accused me of something I hadn't done and I resented the injustice.

'Let's have a look at your childhood,' he says, opening his eyes. 'The wellspring.' His eyes twinkle.

I like that. Lionel is the first person to say this to me, and it is unusual – we didn't 'look at our childhoods' then. *Wellspring*, I love the word. We can look into the wellspring together. I go away to make a list of my early memories. And when I'm home my mum helps me. As ever she's only too keen to look back at the old days with my dad when we were small. She still makes that part of her life all rosy.

I remember Greenbanks, our cottage outside Box in Wiltshire, when I was four. I remember the garden. Mum tells me how I snipped off the flower heads – Dad's best dahlias! I took some scissors from the house and Snip, Snip, Snip. Then, in a moment of pure horror, I snipped off the tip of our cat's ear. Just the tip, but I was left with the piece of silky ear in my hand.

And there's my best friend Mark. We went to Mrs Lyons' kindergarten on the bus. The bus ran over a dog, a golden Labrador, and they lifted it off the road; they left the great lump of the dog in the grass by the road. A live grass snake was being shown at the school, it wasn't slimy but dry and smooth to the touch. Our nanny caught a mouse in the trap, dangled it by the tail, lifted the heavy lid of the range and dropped it into the fire.

I ripped up books at Clare's feeding times, Mum said.

And then there was baby Catherine already. But Mum no longer there. She had gone into the Barrow Hospital in Bristol with a nervous breakdown. It was the time of our evacuation from Box to our grandfather WAF's in Sussex. We never saw Mum and hardly saw Dad, who was always at work. It was a desperately difficult time, he said. Grandpa was away at work in London too. We were kept under our step-grandma's iron thumb. Clare's punishment for tipping her baby sister out of the pram was to be tied to a kitchen chair for a morning; my punishment for wetting the bed was to stay in the gardener's sight all day while everyone else went off to the seaside at Littlehampton. When Dad found out how unhappy we were, he came and took us away on Christmas Eve. We drove away and he stopped to buy a tree and tied it to the roof of the car. I don't know where we ended up that Christmas.

22. Green window

I begin a painting in my studio space at last: a four-foot square canvas of the view through the window. I can't be bothered to make a proper stretcher this time, just nail together the four lengths of wood; the unstretched canvas sags.

A slab of lawn, intensely green, tilted towards the picture plane to fill most of the canvas; the eye directed at the lawn, the rest periphery; shapes of the ornamental trees lined along the top, ragged against a February sky; the whole thing seen through the window. A realistic, objective painting.

How can you paint objectively if you see a different, subjective set of colours? says the Spoiler.

I can, I can. Just look hard, harder than I've ever looked before. Nature will always show something new and unexpected. The blackbirds and starlings feeding on the bright green grass become part of the picture.

The mantra keeps returning: First learn how to paint objectively. Include the studio mess, the nuts and bolts, whatever's there. And that keynote of the Euston Road: keep the mistakes and measuring marks, don't rub them out; they're all part of the process, the history of the work, its integrity. There's a beautiful example of this in *Diary of a Pear* by Euan Uglow, in which we see the pear gradually subside, shrivel and rot as he paints it.

I become obsessed with my window painting, put in a huge number of hours. I keep it going through my depression, won't let it go. I go in at weekends too. On Sunday morning, when the studios are locked, I get in through the window. I actually prefer to work in the studios at the weekend, when there's no one around, when there's no canteen, so this isn't new. And I'm not entirely alone in there. The window has been left open for others too. Some third years, just a couple of months away from their degree shows, are also working weekends. Colin Smith is there. And Skeet with her eyepatch squinting at her perspectives. There's a guy called Andy with whom I argue about rock music over the screens. He can't 'hear' classical music; all music must have 'a rock heartbeat' for it to be true, according to him.

But *Green Window* gets heavier and heavier. The more I put in the more it bogs down. I want that lawn to leap out at me with all spring's brilliance, but it won't. The paint just sinks and dies. Even the glossy blackbirds and irridescent starlings can't bring it back up. And then all the other greens in the gardens behind. The problem with the greens in my picture is they aren't true living greens. I look around. Simon can mix a lifelike green – though since he discovered Giacometti, he hasn't been looking out of the window, and there isn't much green in the life room. I watch the Barefoot Wonder paint. This shaggy golden-haired first-year works with supreme confidence and abandon. Lays it on thick, unmixed, straight from the tin. Doesn't fuss or labour over it. Works for an hour and pads away on his broad bare feet, satisfied. My greens are funny greens, notes off key. In the end that's what they are. I've tried, applied all the theory, but in the end I'm kidding myself. And I'm beating myself senseless here. My Black Dog still has some way to run.

I look at John Magoldrick, a master of colour too, creator of the masterful painting that hangs on Swanpool Street stairs. He disappeared for a year and has turned up at the college again. They've let him back on the course. He has a painting space which he shares with the meticulous sable brush painter Steve. John's usually around on Sundays when Steve isn't there, partly because he doesn't really have anywhere to live. I heard Lionel put him up when he first arrived, then he started to move around from floor to floor, or bush to bush. John is wild-eyed, seems a little mad. He's had a knock on the head, he says, he always says. He paints fast, fluently, like the Barefoot Wonder, but he has stopped painting what's in front of him – the light through a window he once so beautifully caught; the light through the window I'm still trying to catch – and is now working on something called *The Red Man*, some part of himself only he can see. It feels things are going downhill for John quite fast. Sisyphus can't keep on rolling that rock up the mountain; one day he will let it roll back on himself.

There are still weekly drawing trips. What a relief to jump in the college bus with Ray and drive away from the claustrophobic art school. Even if it is a damp grey morning. We explore the upper Fal, an area of quiet muddy tidal creeks, thickly wooded, trees growing right down to the water's edge. There's a graveyard of oil tankers on the main channel. These monster ships have been driven up there and apparently abandoned; you come across one suddenly, a great hulk growing algae, filling the view. We could stop and draw these tankers in the mud. But today we cross the river at King Harry Ferry and drive through remote St Just in Roseland to the coast at the end, find a great empty house there on the water's edge. It's the strangest place, cobwebby, forgotten, something out of Daphne du Maurier's *Vanishing Cornwall*. We leave the gear in the back of the bus and have a day of exploration instead of art. Walk round the derelict gardens, clamber through overgrown hedges to the beach and pick our way along the slimy shore. Then it's back to the canteen.

The canteen! What a nightmare! It's turned itself into a perfect little hell. I walk down the college hill into the thick of it, steer and propel myself in from behind. Ten minutes of eternity in a canteen queue. Sartre's vision of hell: people. Being stuck for ever in a lift with the same people. Or a queue … Hey, I've just come for my lunch for Chrissakes! Let me have some lunch, please! I unglue myself from the wall and inch round … 'Oh he's pale as a ghost today. What can I get you, my lover? Pasty? Saffron cake?' The smiley dinner lady laughs kindly and serves me one of her Cornish pasties stuffed with gravelly mince. You've got to laugh to get through. Let me see, was I going to sit at Pasters' table? I've been wanting to ask him about joining his band. I think I'd like to be the lead singer in his band at the dance. Yes me, the wee tim'rous beastie. Or consider joining a women's table, Lizzie and Carol's, maybe? Just consider it.

Probably, I sat at an easy table that day. The world is divided into easy and difficult tables, and the college canteen is no exception. Paul B's was easy. Paul is a cheery chap from Brum who does painstaking little figurative paintings, realistic like miniature Brueghel, like Hilliard, but not real. Not about the light and texture of the world, I think, but about his own dreams. Unfortunately, I do confuse him with that curious painter Anthony Green, who came to give a talk and whose polygonal paintings of domestic family life I don't get on with at all. Green is still exhibiting these things at the Royal Academy nearly forty years later. I know that Paul will stick with his art too – all he does is his art. He will go on to the RA himself, and I see now that he won the 'Not the Turner Prize' in 2004. So he's still a bastion of that patient, realistic, old-fashioned painting done with fine brushes.

Yes, this is the day I've come out of a Lionel session to babble everything that's in my head to a bewildered, yet amiably (and admirably) still grinning Paul. I often feel as bad after talking to Lionel as I did before. But Paul doesn't seem to mind my yakking on. He says he would happily incorporate a tiny father figure on a Japanese glacier into one of his paintings, or a mother inside a doll's house wardrobe. He's an untroubled person, Paul. But of course he isn't. He's as socially awkward as me. He keeps to himself, works all the time, has few friends. I'm sure he's really glad that I sat down and talked to him. It must work both ways.

23. Help yourself

I don't find Simon in the canteen at all. He doesn't go there for the same paranoid reasons I don't, I will discover years later. Los Paranoias! While I've been labouring with my funny greens, scurrying between my space and the canteen, Simon has been holding out in the life room, plugging away at his new, dark, intense drawings. I go for tea and a cigarette with him (alone I smoke my pipe, in company it's cigarettes) and listen to him pontificate about the existentialist space closing in on us, crushing us, the heaviness of the air. His figures are getting thinner like Giacometti's, as the air closes round and compresses them. They are hard drawings to look at.

This period coincides with the split with one of the loves of his life, the girl who does all the dancing. I won't intrude. One can leave some spaces.

What of the other tutors, the part-timers and occasionally seen? Ron Smith, a small round man in biker's leathers, came bustling round the studios dishing out copies of Mao's *Little Red Book*. He doesn't look at my painting. His life is all politics, the only politics there is at Falmouth. I don't know what kind of work Ron does, and he never talks to me about mine, but he impresses Maoism on me for a while. He gives a passionate, proselytizing lecture: Art for Art's Sake. He wants artists with a purpose and mission in society, eventually leading to the Overthrow and us all becoming Communist artists. I don't have any such mission. I throw away my *Red Book* and sing a line from a 10cc song: Art for art's sake, money for God's sake.

The musician-in-residence, Martin, is an orange man, a follower of Bhagwan Shree Rajneesh. He runs a Dynamic Meditation group. I go once. It's a kind of encounter session.

Encounter groups are setting up everywhere, they are intimately linked with art and art events, with happenings; they're Art with Psychology; they're about the Here and Now. There are five stages to a DM session: with closed eyes, ten minutes of rapid breathing through the nose, which give you a dizzy high; ten minutes of catharsis, where you allow whatever's happening – laughter, shouting, screaming; ten minutes of jumping up and down with arms raised shouting 'hoo'; fifteen minutes of silence and stillness; and fifteen minutes of dancing and celebration.

I will meet Martin later in London, at a party in Highgate which turns out to be full of orange people, and see the creepiness of this cult. By then Bhagwan has become known as 'the sex guru' who lubricates his meditation with sex and owns a fleet of Rolls-Royces; he is eventually indicted in America for poisoning the water supply of Dallas (with salmonella) and deported. He will go round the world being refused entry to country after country, including Britain, and end up in his native Poona, where he dies young.

Peter Redgrove is back from teaching in the States. It's rare to have a poet as writer-in-residence at an art school, and all down to the boldness of the previous Principal. Peter will get himself into plenty of trouble with the current and future college Principals for his 'taking over' of the plastic arts. He is now part of a husband and wife writing partnership with Penelope Shuttle; they have recently published *The Hermaphrodite Album* and are busy writing *The Wise Wound*. He's a large man with his T-shirt, jeans and sandals (whisky flask in back pocket). With his domed forehead and booming voice that can dominate any room, he intimidates me.

But I don't see much of him. He lives somewhere up on the hill and hardly comes into the studios these days. After teaching at the art school for many years, he now has an unofficial counselling role similar to Lionel's. Peter is another Jungian and keeper of dream diaries. He has rescued many a struggling student by showing them writing. In Complementary Studies, like Lionel, he cross-fertilises art with science, mythology and psychology. Simon lives near him. He once took Peter a dream for analysis (the interpretation was premature ejaculation, and he was advised on techniques to master it). Kate, who has a room in Simon's house now, 'in her room writing all the time', is very close to him. I feel I've missed out on Redgrove.

There are some wild stories around. Apparently, in marital crisis in the late 60s, he went on drinking bouts lasting days with the writer D.M. Thomas, and with his way-out analyst John Layard (who also taught at the college). Peter would take his students 'mud-bathing' on the creeks of the Fal. After one evening of late tutorials, conducted in the pub, a group of them went up to Devoran Creek and leapt fully clothed into the tidal mud in the moonlight. It was part of his preoccupation with mud, an obsession which he called the Game and troubled much of his life. He kept it a close secret and was terrified of being found out right up to the end. This is all spelled out now in Neil Roberts' fine new biography *A Lucid Dreamer*. Redgrove's radio play, *Dance of the Putrefact*, broadcast by the BBC in 1975, features immersion in mud. There's a lot of dangerous estuary mud around here.

A hypnotist comes to give a lecture and gets the whole audience to quit smoking. Some achievement for one person standing at the front of the darkened lecture hall to bend thirty people to her will, it seems to me. You have to show willing, go with its flow, she says, or it won't work. I show willing and it works for me – for a day – which I consider to be something of a triumph. The desire to smoke is actually removed – until I stop showing willing. It will be another twenty years before I have that realisation myself and stick to it because I want to, and really quit. I take her address in Torquay with a mind to getting some of my other problems 'hypnotised away' too. It almost worked with nicotine so why not them too? But I don't pursue it. Apathy and inertia win over. The grist to the Dog's mill, of course. It's not in the Spoiler's interest to help you get out of your hole, is it? He'll keep you down there with a padlocked grating on top for as long as he can.

I reinstate my pipe and fumigate my room. The pungency of tobacco! Everywhere smells of tobacco in the seventies, all the pubs, cafés, cinemas, offices, public places – how sensitised we've all become in the short time since the change of law; we ex-smokers must be the worst, we can detect a cigarette from a mile off, get a whiff through the open car window as we pass the hospital exits where the lucky smokers still congregate in their hospital gowns. At Falmouth, in my room, I create a dreadful fug. Jam the pipe in my gob when I start to paint and there it remains. When I become aware of the stink it only makes me light up again for a fresh bit of smoke.

One morning I light up in the library (amazing to be smoking a pipe in a library) and Lionel wanders in.

'Didn't know you smoked a pipe?'

'Yes.' I blush.

'Is it the smell? How did you get on with *The Outsider*?'

The writer Colin Wilson, who recently moved down to Cornwall, has been to give a talk. He described how his book had come to him while he was hitching up the M1 and got stuck at the St Neot's interchange in Leicestershire: he was an outsider to society! He called his epiphany the 'St Neot's Margin'. I think of myself as a bit of an outsider in a resentful and hateful way, but he seems to relish it. It's his strength. That's what Lionel has been thinking too.

'Outsiders aren't such bad things to be,' he says. 'I have Colin's book somewhere if you'd like to borrow it. His notion of "peak experiences" is most interesting. You know, I reread your story of a day of hell, walking around the town afraid and lost, and that could be regarded as a peak experience. We've been catching some of your childhood memories, haven't we? And fascinating they are. You could try making a bit of a story out of those as well. The run-over dog. That nice smooth snake in your kindergarten. And goodness, the box of bullets from the war you and your friend found dumped under the bridge! We'll talk more next time. Don't *entirely* give up on the dreams, though. I always think dreams are the true key, as I've said before.'

Lionel meanders out of the library without looking at any books. He only came in because he smelt the smoke.

Before going to see him I should work out what to say. Help myself. Save him an hour of roundabout talking. But I don't. The Spoiler prefers lethargy. Hey, *you* can't be master of the situation, you must be its slave. I want to run after Lionel and tell him now … but I don't. I don't *know* what I want to say yet. It's easier to stick to the arrangement. See him next week. But I kick and rail at myself for doing nothing. I never consider he might *want* me to wait until the next appointment, that there's a point to it, a rhythm and routine he's trying to instil; when I will be ready for him.

When I do tell him the above, offering an apology, he responds typically, always differently. 'You don't have to write things down if you don't want to. You just need to think *why* you don't want to. Which is why dreams are so good. They show us things, if we can only reach the code. They are here to help us.'

'Dreams are a kind of self-help course, then?'

'Exactly,' Lionel says fervently.

Hypnosis, Dynamic Meditation, salvation through Mao … There's a lot of this self-help around. There are Encounters. One day Leo comes through the studios clicking her fingers. She pops her head into my space and tells me about a Psychokinesis encounter group I might be interested in. I'm still working on *Green Window*. Let's say I'm not attacking it for a change, but seeing how dark the white window frame appears against the sky – a deep blue or purple. The only way the window can be lightened is by whitening the sky.

Laurie from sculpture is running the encounter group. I know Laurie from the pub, where he props up the bar, tucking away pints and chain-smoking. He always has time to talk about the meaning of art. He knows about such things as Christo's amazing wrapping up of buildings and hanging curtains across a canyon in the Colorado desert; sculpture on a new huge scale, environmental art. He shares some interests here with existential Thom. One of Laurie Burt's own pieces, a bronze that looks like an old flatiron, is called, marvellously, *Small meaningless object created for the tactile appreciation of nothing*. (It was bought by Falmouth Art Gallery in 2007.)

'What's a Happening, Laurie?'

'A Happening? Mm, a live Installation. Anything you want to name.'

The truth of it is there's room for all kinds of art, myriad art forms. Room for Gilbert and George, and Anne Bean, and wacky Bruce Lacey, and for all the traditional painting from nature too. They can all co-exist. That's what I wanted to tell De Gruyter back in Reading.

It's extraordinary how kind, thoughtful Laurie smokes and smokes. I can't believe how he has to light up another straightaway. My history teacher at school was a 60-a-day man. He couldn't 'last' and would slip out to the corridor for a fag mid-lesson; his next smoke was built into the structure of the lesson. Then there was Fitz at Reading, his double whammy of pipe alternating with cigarettes through art history seminars – no need to leave the room. I do quite well myself, though I'm not in the same league as these guys. Looking online now, it's even more extraordinary to find that Laurie Burt has survived those zillions of cigarettes, is still alive and a practising artist at 88.

I go along to see what his Psychokinesis is about. We are a small group. Leo is there as ever in her leopardskin. Laurie wheezes his way through an exposition of the self-help system of telekinesis. Basically, it's a 'mind over matter' thing. Moving objects with the mind. The spoonbender Uri Geller is a well-known exponent. I don't, and still don't, believe a word of that spoon-bending malarkey but am happy to be led by Leo through a 'guided daydream', which I write down. It's about putting yourself into a place in your mind and being there.

> Both places are home, one in Wiltshire, one in Somerset, I can't decide which. Decide I'm in Wiltshire, standing by the river near my father's house. The wooded valley sides rise sharply on either side. I cross to the road which runs down one side and begin walking down to the village. A bus. It starts as a single deck green country bus and changes to a London red double-decker, then back to the green. It stops and I stand by the door while a crowd of people pour out. Mostly old people, no individual faces. I follow the road into Castle Combe, meet an old man in a cloth cap on a bicycle. He doesn't materialise fully, is gone. As I pass the bridge at the edge of the village, the green bus comes again. Lots of blurred faces on it. Colonel Birch is standing beside me with his dog straining at the leash. He waves and grins. His grinning face freezes like a photograph, turns into a hollow mask, fades. There's a wrought-iron gate, which I open, and I walk up an asphalt path to a white suburban house. I'm afraid of who's inside. I knock. The door is opened by a young woman in a 40s white mac and hairstyle – an actress, someone I know. It's my mother when she was young, the face

> of a photo, and we stand in silence. She has to break the silence, recognize me. She doesn't, she picks up a suitcase and leaves. I follow her on to the bus, get in behind and sit in the empty seats at the back. Then I move up next to her and finally hold her hand and feel better. She takes a Kleenex from her bag which turns into an ice cream.

These dreamlike images rest unreferred to in my diary – they seem like the seeds of a poem now. I don't go back to Psychokinesis but among the reading list I take away with me is Arthur Janov's *The Primal Scream*, a cult book of the time, which will have a powerful influence over me. Not intellectually, more of a punch below the belt. It's about how much of our adult life relates back to early childhood, how we all need to get back there at some stage and, well, have a good primal scream.

'Did you get to Peter's talk?' says Lionel. '*Fascinating*.'

We are half way through the spring term now, how slow it's been, and Peter Redgrove has given his extraordinary talk on *The Wise Wound*, the book he and his wife Penny are writing about menstruation and the moon. He talked about the effect of the monthly lunar cycle on women, the tides in the female body. 'As a woman is more than fifty per cent water,' he said, 'it's evident she'll have her own internal tides: high and low, spring and neap.' He said something like, When you're next with your wife/lover/girlfriend, ask if you can look inside her vagina. Deep inside her you will see a crescent moon.

Can this be true? I don't believe him. But I don't know. He means the cervix, doesn't he? Is it moon-shaped? I would like to see that but I don't have anyone to ask. Still no one. Actually I wonder about the practicalities too. When I'm with someone, such intimate investigations hardly seem possible. There's no real, lasting relationship like that on my horizon. It seems my life will only ever be a series of short flings now and 'May I look at your cervix?' isn't on the cards.

'Bad for the digestion to eat with your legs crossed,' says Pasters passing my table where I'm eating alone. 'Did they teach you nothing at home?' Indeed, all the tension of being alone in the teeming canteen has been squeezed into my crossed legs. I'm braving it out, having a decent lunch of pie and chips. But it was good of Pasters. He has moved out of Swanpool now but is always friendly when we meet in college. Still seems to like me, however miserable I get. I can't see why. He's such a comedian and extravert, my opposite. 'You're a piss artist, Pasters, talking to a snail in its shell, a wood louse in a curl,' I might have told him.

'Join us?' he says.

I look across to his intimidating table with Leafy, Johnnie and Derek. Lionel says that apathy is all the internal aggression unable to get out.

'Okay.'

They are fomenting rebellion. Art is getting too serious for its own good. It's up its own arse. So precious and ivory tower with its private painting spaces.

'Craft is what it's all about,' says Johnnie. 'Making useful things. Beautiful useful things. And keeping traditions alive. Pottery, weaving, smithing.'

'What do you you reckon, Froy?'

Maybe I say 'Beauty follows function follows form …'

But I don't do that. This time I stay put, say, 'Thanks, but I'll stick here. Must be getting back to work.' I uncross the legs that have betrayed me and take a gulp of scalding tea. I come to my rescue. Nothing wrong with sitting alone to think about things, is there? When I'm painting I get lost in myself all the time. I only came to the canteen out of necessity and of course I don't want to talk to anyone. Don't want to break the spell. I *want* to stay inside myself. That's the whole point. So I'm not going to join some blokey table like drummer Pasters' and while away the afternoon. I finish up and scuttle back to the studio to reengage with the painting of ghastly greens.

Then I pass him practising with his band. Pasters, Leafy and Judy are in the lecture hall playing raucously. It's a weekend afternoon, which only makes matters worse. *Why are you alone at the weekend? Join in.* This rough, loud stuff is so attractive. I want to join them. I'm gonna get up on that little stage and prance around as the lead singer (they already have Judy as their lead singer). I'm not the quiet bassist at the back, or the drummer like Pasters, loud at the back, but the singer right out at the front of the stage. That's me.

'That's me, Lionel! Quiet, sensitive, depressed JF!'

Lionel grunts. He isn't very interested. He's thinking: if that's what JF wants to do, then he can do it for himself. I'm not going to put my energies there. These little mountains we have to climb for ourselves.

'Well, I hope you do get up on that stage, John. Any new memories or dreams?'

24. Some way to run

It isn't over yet. There's a black hole after lunch. By mid afternoon I'm making another furtive escape from my studio space. I take the hole-in-the-hedge route back to my room. On the way I have a clear image of a drawing I'll do as soon as I get in: the road in front of me, the tarmac of the steep hill that's in my face every day; its texture, the thick line-paint, a manhole; a crooked arrow left or right, a straight ahead arrow, an elongated Give Way triangle in perspective. Quite abstract. As I near Swanpool Street, the image fades. By the time I'm home, my slippery mind has escaped again. Like some prankster playing tricks on myself, I have reprogrammed myself to go charging back to the studio with plans for all the things I will do there.

But I don't go back. I get off that merry-go-round and do the drawing *here*, on my knees, working on the floor. By evening, after a couple of hours of scribbling in soft pencil and chalk, the pitch-black mood has gone. Almost gone. It will come back, but I can always get back at it too. I make out a fresh programme of work:

Paint 3-4 hours daily in a steady, organized way. Gradually accumulate skill and knowledge, producing simple modest objects without pretension and without having to prove anything to anyone (ideal self).

Back in the studio, the green window painting isn't that bad, is it? It has *some* good points.

Lionel talks about opposites. He is keen on the great dualities. Light and dark, open and closed, courage and fear. Fear isn't necessarily a bad thing. We can explore fear. My self-doubt, a form of timidity, is as valuable as another's self-confidence. Everything has its good side, he says. The very worst feelings from the bottom of the pit point to their opposite. This is all deeply encouraging. If I can get out of this by understanding, not by squashing with pills, things might be as good as they have been bad.

'Hairy legs, you say?' says Lionel. He eggs me on, wants me to come out with it. I've said I can't stand women with hairy legs. He wanted me to say something outrageous and I have. 'And armpits?' he probes. I suddenly remember my mother saying the same about men with hairy chests while we watched a bare-chested James Bond in bed with Miss Honey – I shouldn't know this, Mum! You shouldn't have been telling me this. Actually, it's swung the other way now. Underarm hair, for example, is attractive if it's soft and long, not shaved stubble.

Now he leans towards me, face contorting into a frightful grimace. 'With me it's enormous breasts. I'm sorry, I know this is absolutely awful of me, but they give me the horrors.'

He catches my eye and we both burst out laughing.

'Christ, Lionel!'

'I know. I know. It's so awful of me. Makes me such a shit,' he says, while the tears of relief run down his cheeks. 'It's the threat, isn't it? We're both scared shitless. You're scared of the man in the woman, I'm just terrified of a surfeit of milk!'

'You're very thin, Lionel. Could do with building up,' I say and my sudden audacity surprises me.

'Yes, I am. Much too thin. Thank you, thank you for that.'

No, it isn't over yet, still has a bit more to run. And time, art school time, is frittering away. 'God, depression's such a waste of time!' complains elegant Lydia, the posh theatrical girl in the first year, whom I'm pleased to discover is a fellow sufferer. I'm not the only one. But I only tell myself that because everyone does. It's the thing people say when you're low, along with: Pull your socks up, Keep your pecker up and Rome wasn't built in a day. None of which is much comfort. You're still the one in the

Cohen song, lying supine under the skylight while an hour goes by and you haven't moved your hand.

I find *The Savage God* by A. Alvarez and devour it. Perhaps it's one of those books doing the rounds. Certainly good material for the angst-filled student: all the ways you can top yourself.

Without looking out a copy now, one method has stuck in my mind as the perfect suicide, well, a neat one, anyway. This guy, maybe he was American, went out to the cliffs by Land's End with a bottle of whisky (some sleeping pills too). At this westernmost point he wedged himself precariously into the clifftop and watched the sun sink into the west, sipping his whisky until, sozzled, numb, he at last dropped off into the ocean. Oblivion, peace, painless, clean. That's the way to go. Not like those silly 'How did he die?' quiz games they play at the pub, which often involve suicide methods: there's a pool of water, a rope and a body. And no relation at all to my grandfather Teddy's suicide with a beam and kicked box in his garage.

Of course what immediately presents itself with these perfect-death fantasies is the mess left behind. Who sees it? Who clears it up? In my scenario it's important to drop directly into the sea from the clifftop and not end up on the rocks. A child might find your mangled corpse, a young boy out hunting in the rockpools of Land's End as I have done. Someone went into the garage at Rottingdean and found Teddy hanging. So what about the ones you leave behind? Your family, your friends? They mightn't see the body but they'll know about it in the end. An extension of the cliff-jump suicide has me being dragged out to sea and never found, eaten by sharks. I don't know about 'closure'. The body must be found, and probably seen, the terrible uncertainty of not knowing cleared, the course of events established, to allow for the grieving process. I don't know any of this; there have been no deaths in my immediate family since I was born. My family would be upset – wouldn't they? They might even blame themselves in some way. The 'rational and existential' suicide soon starts to unravel at the seams. We can't leave this world without touching others. It's our salvation in a way.

Lionel asks about my maternal grandfather Teddy's suicide. Teddy, whose WW1 medals Granny Betty gave me. How old was Mum at the time? Was she witness? No, she wasn't but the way she always told it, or screamed it, when we were kids, made it seem she had been a little girl, coming home to find her daddy dead. She didn't. She was twenty-seven at the time, living in Leeds, married to our father. But apparently she did find a drop of blood on the garage floor (blood from hanging?) which shocked her terribly. Her father had indeed entered a terrible fit of depression, got himself some rope, and did the business. *Strangulation by hanging himself in garage at* 37 *Eley Crescent, Rottingdean on* 2*nd May* 1951 *while the balance of his mind was disturbed* it says on the death certificate, a truly horrifying document. It had been Granny Betty who found him and sawed through the rope with a carving knife.

'It was shell shock, Lionel. From the trenches of the Somme. Teddy had it for the rest of his life. Neurasthenia, they called it and gave him a small disability pension. He was never able to hold down a job again. They gave him medals and then left him to it. He lived with his battle dreams for another thirty years until he was sixty-one.'

'Your poor mother, and grandmother. I'm most terribly sorry,' Lionel murmurs.

'Anything new this week? Anything we can pin? Anything more from the child?' he says.

What really seem to be helping are my confessions. It's such a relief to be able to say things. Lionel helped clear guilt over masturbation when I first went to see him – 'Go on, have a good wank!' – and since then we've discovered where that might have originated. It was way back when I was five or six, when I was busy with myself quite openly in the armchair – it was the time when I had just been separated from my mother – and my first stepmother Corinne saw me. She didn't seem upset by it but my father was. In cold fury he sent me to my room. He was angrier than I'd ever seen him and I didn't understand why. I stayed in my room for hours reading my *Eagle* comic but still Daddy didn't come up to explain. It was Corinne who showed heart and eventually brought me my tea.

'So you went out and snipped off his best dahlias!' cries Lionel.

I remind him this was a year or two earlier, but I know what he means. There was a war going on between me and my father when I was six, a war over my mother.

There are more things. Early childhood memories are appearing all the time, as though they are freeing themselves. It's these hidden things I want to tell Lionel. I tell him about bedwetting, the first person I've told after Lise. And of course he isn't in the least surprised. From the way he talks, wetting the bed must be the commonest complaint in the world – I'm so glad this 'sin' can be talked about these days. It's out in the open, on TV. There's absolutely nothing *wrong* with it at all. Nothing to feel that awful *guilt* about. The victim needs *help*.

And I tell him that Corinne was the first woman I had erotic feelings for. Sunbathing with her on the balcony of my father's big house in Bath, I became conscious of her body, the sleek black swimsuit and what might lie underneath it, her tanned legs and arms with their fine black hairs glistening with olive oil.

'And you are upset by women with hairy legs,' Lionel says.

What all this seems to be about – obviously, I can say now but at the time I was astonished to discover it – is the early disappearance of my mother at the age of four or five, and the appearance of a stepmother who became my mother. But who wasn't my mother, and with whom I could have no real physical contact at all. My sisters disappeared to live, separately, with Granny Betty and a nanny. Then my mother remarried and I had a new stepfather, Frank. They lived in a new town, and I went there, reunited with my sisters again. A new family! But ah, then I was shipped off to a boarding school, where I wet the bed with a vengeance.

'I should think so! Boarding school! Public school, they have the nerve to call it!' Lionel rages, waving his arms.

Lionel has things to say about public schools and I must say I enjoy this rant as much as anything we have spoken about. He abhors them. He had a lousy time at his. His friend Lindsay Anderson did too, and he made a wonderful film about it. We discuss *If* with relish. How we enjoyed the final conflagration scene when the kids blow the school to hell. We share memories of beating – children being hit with sticks – the horror of the long sadistic beating scene in the gym.

'Seen John Magoldrick around much?' Lionel sighs. 'Who's going to look after him now? Apparently he's taken some drugs and made it all worse.'

Poor John Magoldrick, another head case for Lionel, like me, no, much worse off than me. But I've been to that edge and seen over ... I put together the pieces of his life I know. He arrived at Swanpool Street looking for a room last September. 'I've had a bang on the head,' he said. He had lived in my room in his first year with a Chinese girl; he painted the wonderful picture that hangs on the stairs. Then he took a year off, disappeared, as Mrs Birch put it. He took LSD in London – the bang on the head –'woke up' in a mental hospital, discharged himself, and hitched away from London not knowing where he was going. Arrived in Birmingham. Hitched again. Amazingly, he said, the car brought him back to Falmouth.

He has no parents. His foster parents shipped him off to boarding school. Out of the way. They washed their hands of him. Was this the case with me? Was I really sent to boarding school to be out of the way? My father went to boarding school and so did his father before him, ergo so should I, is perhaps the answer.

Lionel cries out, 'I'm sorry but that's *exactly* what those schools are all about. They're just conveniences to get us out of parenting.'

One more early memory, just one. Because they pop up for Lionel, as he intends them to. It arrived in the Swanpool Street kitchen while I was frying some eggs for my tea. It's a Proustian taste and smell. Three years ago Granny Helen told me that the world was divided between Proust-lovers and Proust-haters. Now I know I'm one of the former. I fried the eggs in olive oil and left them in the pan longer than usual, so the edges of the whites crisped and burnt and I had to scrape them out. At home in the cupboard under the dresser, therefore no longer used, was an individual frying pan, small, dented, with Bakelite double handles, which had been used to fry eggs in olive oil in our first house at Box, when I was four years old. The smell and the taste of these crispy egg whites was exactly the same; I was taken straight back to when I was living there with my sisters and Mum had already gone.

These were pre-Elizabeth David days when culinary olive oil was hardly available in the UK. You had to buy it in small medicinal quantities from the chemist. My father, who hadn't gone, was very advanced in this respect. I remember going with him to a special shop in Bath to buy a huge tin which 'had to last and cost the earth'. The tin was Italian, covered with ornate lettering, and so big it would have to be kept on the kitchen floor. Then we went to a pub where I had crisps with the salt wrapped in a blue paper twist inside and a small bottle of the most delicious orange juice.

'I loved the crispiness of those egg whites,' I say. I think I'm feeling better.

Lionel says, 'Mmm, can taste them myself. As we were saying before, you could try putting some of these very early memories into a story. Start with the house in Box. Write in the third person if you want. Might help. Might be another strategy.'

I go back to my room and write down all I can remember from the cottage on the edge of the common, my friend Mark Fry, going to Kindergarten. It becomes a short story about John and Mark's adventure in the woods when the farmer's dog gets loose and terrorizes the neighbourhood. It's the first short story I write in my adult life. And the memories keep coming. I've never really stopped remembering. Much of what I recover in my weekly sessions with Lionel will go into my childhood memoir 70 *Waterloo Road*. As I said there, it's largely because I dredged for these memories with Lionel so soon after my childhood, at the age of twenty-two, that I have them at all.

25. The longing

Pasters's friend Johnnie of the big black moustache brings two gorgeous girls to the house one day. He seems to live here on and off. Johnnie is rugged and rangy, attractive to women, I'd say, the kind of guy I'd like to be. The girls, Babs and Françoise, one dark-curled, one with blonde ringlets, are prospective foundation students down from London. I don't know what happens to Françoise but dark Jewish Babs comes back with Johnnie that night and stays, and next morning they come down to the kitchen reeking of sex. How sharp that sex-smell can be. Babs goes off to find her friend and Johnnie proceeds to complain about the positions she put him into. Complain! Maybe I've missed the point and really he's just showing off.

Diary: *Craving, longing, every fibre in my being aching. To touch, feel, be warm, close. Is it for love too, or just the animal? It's animal now, after beer. Something must happen soon or I'll burst. There's been a buildup over the past few days. Everything intense, an awareness of people, tiny details. The things about which I'm usually oblivious are everywhere, staring me in the face. I know it's all frustration and desire, a distortion, but that doesn't help matters.*

Lionel has talked about Wilhelm Reich's Orgone Energy Accumulator – the 'Orgasmatron', as Woody Allen calls it. Size of a telephone box, lined with metal, insulated with steel wool (you get hot in there). A magical box, Reich says, charged up with the life force, concentrated with 'orgone energy', which dissolves repressions, treats cancer, radiation sickness … Einstein tested it for Reich but refuted these claims. Many have praised it though, lived by it: Norman Mailer, J.D. Salinger, Saul Bellow, Allen Ginsberg, Jack Kerouac, Sean Connery. William Burroughs achieved a spontaneous 'no hands' orgasm in his. For me, the promise of release of tension, the curative power of orgasm, seems a marvellous panacea. I'd get in there for that. Wild and wacky Wilhelm Reich might have been, but he had known Freud and escaped the Nazis, who burned his books. He reached America only to be hounded again for his 'fraudulent claims' and have his books burned there too, six tons of them, and be imprisoned. He had a heart attack after a year in prison and died just before his parole.

I'm okay with the pub now. I go there to celebrate a day's painting. I go when I haven't spoken to anyone all day. There's a good crowd at the Summerhill, a crowd of piss artists, we like to call ourselves. Yeah, we artists have to get pissed ... We stay until closing time, hoping for a lock-in but never getting one. One night we go for a winter swim; we all troop off to dunk ourselves in the sea at Gyllyngvase Beach, and it isn't that cold or doesn't seem so with the alcohol coursing through. One night a poet with a shaved head (maybe it was Molly Parkin) gives a piss-artist reading full of f- and c-words at the pub. I haven't heard so many profanities in a public reading and enjoy their blunt power. Kate is in the audience. She's writing masses now.

This time after closing time, some of us – not Kate – stagger down Jacob's Ladder and head for a party 'at Ivan's'. We cross the market square, and then on up the hill on the other side, to a new part of town for me. It's open house at Ivan's parents' house. Ivan isn't at the art school; he's just left school and isn't a student yet. His presence flickers back to me: smallish, lively, funny, playing the ukelele; he's that wonderful thing, a natural musician. He has a girlfriend with the lovely name of Julia Darling who's on the foundation course. Ivan and Julia don't stay long in Falmouth, but go up to art school in Newcastle. Julia will earn a high reputation with her poetry, short stories and novels, and die tragically young of breast cancer.

It's the thing to dress up at Ivan's, be experimental, in drag or a combination, a bit of AC/DC for the dance. All part of the coming out of the early 70s, the sparkly ostentatious boy/girl glam rock thing as exemplified by David Bowie and Marc Bolan. It isn't gay, or consciously so – the word itself is still hardly in use down here; there are no openly gay people at the college. Instead, there are dressers-up, latter-day hippies in exotic silks and velvets, and cross-dressers – we don't use that word either; we just say 'drag'. There are women in coats and tails, and men with beards in skirts.

I'm like a Moody at the party. I'm at their house in Poplar I was invited to but never went. I'm with the scandalous pair at the gallery opening in the King's Road, wearing one black and one white shoe. With them in Germany in a famous *Sunday Times* colour supplement picture of 1974. Sparkly platform shoes on paint-spattered steps. I'm among the beautiful, pouting, raunchy girls like Rod, the only guy left in the band, singing with him 'Help Me Through the Night' the best you've ever heard it.

On the way home I'm 'outrageous', crawling over the bonnet of a Rolls-Royce parked in the market square, which has the misfortune to be in my way.

Colin Smith, the true star painter at the college, now going to the Royal College, was at the party and we talked about the difference between being in London at the centre of things and stuck down here on England's toe. Colin said life on the toe was a lot cushier. Half-drunk when I arrived, I proceeded to get rat-arsed with him. Though he's a tall dark swarthy type with a piratical earring, his small mouse voice is always a surprise. Yes, I could go and live in the East End of London, get a studio in Wapping with him, I reckon. He lives on a houseboat upriver at Penryn at the moment and can't paint his large canvases on the boat; I'm lucky to have my room at Swanpool Street to stretch out in.

26. Mother

I'm half out of the dumps. Climbing back up. Lionel gets me to talk about my mother. He's the first person to do this, as he was the first to open out my childhood. Lionel wakes me up to her.

She provokes different moods in him, one minute full of sympathy – when I told him about her shell-shocked father's suicide – and the next, well, exasperation. He surprises me by suggesting that Frank is too soft on her. He allows her too much, indulges her, and this is partly why she behaves so badly.

He doesn't sleep with her now, though. He's in a separate room at the end of the corridor. My room.

But he looks after her. And she needs him. She couldn't manage without him. She's never had a job, my mum, apart from Carlisle in the war. She's hardly been out in the world fending for herself. She's lived at home all the time, had children, got ill.

Alarmingly, Lionel tells me that I hate my mother. In order to love her again I must cut her up into pieces, and examine each piece by looking for memories of her. Good can only come from the very worst. 'Plants grow out of shit.'

I hate him for saying this.

But he wants me to complain about her. So I do. 'She's always ill, wrapped up in herself. The ill always are. They can't spare energy for other people.'

Now I'm the bruised and scathing teenager who can't bear having a loony mother, who shuts his mum away in a corner of his mind. Drinking, shoplifting, pill-popping Mum. All those pills they give her on the NHS; every time they come up with a new psychotic drug, they give it to her to try. Migraine Mum – she still gets bad migraines despite all the pills. Stay-at-home Mum who doesn't have a job but doesn't do any housework or cooking either. Frank does all that. Frank, the opposite, the rock and anchor, the worker, carer, home doctor; the cook, cleaner, washerwoman; all of these things. It's true, all true. She's asphyxiating and I just have to get away from her.

As I rant against my useless mother to Lionel, I feel my indignation rise in her defence. Anger struggles with bruises. She isn't all bad. She's good at preparing grapefruit in segments, sugared and soaked; she never forgets your birthday; she has a lovely laugh, when she can laugh. Of course she isn't all bad. No one is, almost no one. And in spite of myself, I see now I'm rooting for her. On her side. Like her. Whatever I say or do I am close to her.

These endless waves, the crashing rocks, the shingle-sucking undertow of my mother. I wish I could be clearer.

In my room I get out some of her letters, which I've always kept for reasons that should be clear by now. That eight-pager to my grim room in Turnpike Lane. *Just tired, NOT drun.* Believe her. Just very worked up; maybe it was just some new pills. *It would be so nice if you could climb through the window or something on my birthday.* Yes, I could do that. I imagine her now, padding round the house in her slippers with the radio, listening to Wogan and Jimmy Young. Another letter, one to her mother, which Granny Betty gave to me with a hard stare. It's from the autumn of 1970 when I've just left home and am working on the Christmas chocolates counter in John Lewis, Bristol. 'John craves affection.' she writes, 'and could one day make a very nice husband and father – but he'll have to get down to brass tacks sooner or later. I don't want such good material to turn into a drifter.' I clutch at these words of concern for me. Then see: *some of us never find ourselves* and laugh at this little joke she's made at her own expense.

I would have liked a bit of help from her. Some empathy when I was right down at the bottom, which after all she knows plenty about. Yes, a bit of support for a start. She was always the patient making the demands. It was always about me making allowances for her. I can smile now but later on, years later, when I'm more settled and she still isn't, she will actually ask me to be her psychiatrist. And though the idea fills me with horror, I do consider it in a way. I try to see things from her point of view. The misunderstood, the misfit. It's true she doesn't fit easily into small-town Wellington life; she talks about London all the time because that's where she would like to live. So she gets all she can out of Clare being at the Slade, she goes to *Last Tango* at the local fleapit, she gets drunk in her frustration, and funny things happen to her in the chip shop queue. She may not fit so well with Frank after all.

Lionel raises these questions for which I don't have answers. Why is she in a state all the time? Why always an ill mother, a special case? When did it start? Was it with my father? Was it more to do with having us children? And have I inherited this depression from my mother who got it from her father? I will later realise that I am an inheritor to some extent of what she calls the 'family curse'. I do have the tendency.

Mum will continue to rage until her menopause. And it's during her menopause in the early eighties that the real climax comes, the mother humdinger of it all. Then it will be said by more than one psychiatrist, as they continue to pump her full of the latest drugs, that her troubles have been much to do with child-bearing; she's a woman who shouldn't have had four kids. And when *that* is finally over, things will eventually settle down in her mind. And they do, mostly, in the end.

I tell Lionel about a big bad day of rampage in the summer of 1974, when I was at home waiting to come down to Falmouth. I've hardly made the connection until now that it might be my mother's behaviour, her ups and downs, that are starting to affect me in a way they didn't use to. I *arrived* here in a mess, on Valium, escaping from a mother who was having a ripsnorter of a summer.

'An astonishing day,' Lionel agrees. 'I hope the little one's going to manage all right. Do you think she will?'

'Sarah? I don't know. We went to the hospital to visit Mum last summer.'

'Tell me about that.'

I close my eyes in Lionel's room and revisit my mother in Tone Vale Hospital with Frank and Sarah. I've only ever been there twice, the first time when I was thirteen. In fact both visits were rather similar – I was a child visiting my mum in the loony bin.

Sarah and I picked a bunch of her favourite sweet peas from the garden. I sat with Sarah in the back seat of the car – comfort, solidarity – and Frank drove us through the long winding country lanes. He went every day, after school, at weekends. 'I've done this journey 100 times,' he'd say. In all Mum went to Tone Vale seven times, forty-four weeks, and Frank visited over three hundred times; he gave up going daily in the end. 'It's a gloomy old Victorian pile,' he warned. The clipped yew hedges reminded me of my boarding school and cast a little chill, a dread of being left on the steps while my parents drove away: see you at Christmas! See you at Easter! Her room was on the ground floor on a long disinfected corridor.

She was ready to go out, impatient. Frank said she wasn't always; sometimes she couldn't face going out at all. But today she could hardly stand still. When she tried to be still, her feet continued to knead the floor like a cat. From the drugs. She put on her jacket and dark glasses. The zipped, black-and-white striped fur jacket, her 'ski jacket', was posh from London, from when she was with my father, and she'd hung on to it. And a silk square for her head, which she always wore when out. She had dozens of these scarves at home. When she found a good source she bought them all up. We couldn't afford it. Frank grumbled. Buying 'unnecessary things' had always been one of the ways she got into trouble with him.

We walked back along the corridor, past all the numbered doors. The doors had no handles on the inside. 'Like police cars,' she said.

Padded rooms. Straitjackets. Shock Treatment. We grew up aware of these things because of her father, Teddy. He had all that during the thirties.

She didn't want to go for a drive today, just a walk in the grounds would be enough. Frank, who came every day, said he'd stay in the car; he had a book. So Sarah and I took her to the patients' gardens and their little zoo. We had to cross a wooden footbridge, guide our mum across the slippery planks. This sort of thing was always a palaver. There was the business of her heels, she had the wrong shoes on. She wobbled on her heels with her weight, might get a heel stuck between the planks. She'd fallen in this situation before now. But we got her safely across and went to look at the cages. There were rabbits and guinea pigs for Sarah. There were exotic Golden and Lady Amherst's pheasants – the last time I was here I'd spent the time poking through the wire of their cages trying to retrieve one of their lovely discarded tail feathers; I was still quite keen to do this. We looked at the pond with its ducks, a big brown Muscovy duck with her ducklings. Sitting on the grass by the murky pond, Mum talked about Jemima Puddleduck and Jeremy Fisher.

She talked about getting back to Art Therapy in the hospital. The teacher was a sympathetic woman too, and Mum might be able to help with the teaching soon. She rambled on, garrulous, sounding relaxed, quite happy in a way.

She said an odd thing, a memory from when she was with Dad. 'Your father didn't like Art Therapy, the whole idea of it.

Everybody trying to express themselves as though they were Van Goghs. He said that was where art had gone wrong, with the Expressionists. All the Expressionists, he dumped them in one basket. Of course, he was so terribly Classical. Cézanne and Poussin. Of course I like Cézanne too – even if he did have an awful time with women – but I like Van Gogh too. I've always loved Vincent.'

'Personally,' she went on, 'I agree with the teacher here. You've got to make a mess to start. The more mess the better.'

The drugs did funny things with Mum. Sometimes they made her fuzzy, sometimes quite lucid – that sharp remark about Cézanne and women. She hadn't had any shock treatment yet. She'd be telling us about it, its ghastliness, the going under and coming back.

ECT. Electroconvulsive Therapy. We grew up with people talking about shock treatment because Teddy had had it. A really barbaric business then – you've seen the films, that grainy old hospital bed scene with electrodes, rubber bung in the mouth, white coats around the bed to hold the patient down ... the switch ... the convulsing body ... Of course it isn't quite like that now, there are anaesthetics, muscle relaxants. It isn't agony but you can still feel the jolts. You can still get burns.

Yet she agreed to have Shock. Or everyone went on at her so long she was persuaded. She tried to look on the positive side. Ludovic Kennedy had it voluntarily, she said, because it worked for him, it lifted him out of his depression almost magically; he would rather have the electricity than the drugs. She tried to be positive but she was afraid. Sometimes she begged Frank to take her home, now. Now.

The results of Mum's ECT were startling and immediate, not like the drugs at all. She became loud and full of laughter. Her natural laugh rang unnaturally. When Frank cracked a joke at mealtimes she laughed and laughed. Frank wrote to me: *Mum is blooming. The treatment seems to have had an almost magical effect on her.* This buoyant mood lasted for some time, a season, and in that way it was perfect. The only problem was memory. She lost a chunk of her short-term memory. But it came back in the end, pieced itself together again, or *nearly* all of it, she said. She didn't actually remember much of the business itself after the electrodes went on.

It was getting late. We had to go. Frank wanted to get back to cook the supper. Granny Betty would be needing her supper too. We went back over the footbridge to the car and left her behind.

'Thank you,' says Lionel.

Granny Betty must have visited her too with Frank. Well, of course she did if Frank went every day. I have a note Mum wrote to her in Tone Vale. Slight and lucid.

T.V.
19/7/75
9.20 p.m.

My dear Mother,

It was lovely to see you both again so soon. I am just about falling asleep … although I am nervous of those nightmares again and can't remember if there is another round of pills to keep awake for!

Much love Anne. xxx

p.s. It is a v. good orange stick – thanks again.

*

Lionel wants me to talk about my other mother too, Corinne, my stepmum, who took over when Mum disappeared into Barrow

Hospital when I was six. Corinne the talented sculpture student who'd won some West of England sculpture prize. Corinne has always been taboo. Everything to do with her has this air of secrecy.

When her letters came to Wellington, to Colham, the pale blue envelopes with Kent postmarks addressed to any or all of us, they filled me with horror and dread. They were bare and shocking. They were crazy riddles. There was such urgency to them. They fascinated me, were connected to me in some way. I kept a few of them and came across them when I was researching this.

I show Lionel one of Corinne's letters, explaining that the date at the top isn't the date it was written, but the date it's about.

20th January 1963
I heard 'Mama'. I thought it was midnight, awoke. Maria was holding out her arms
to me and the light was streaming from her eyes.
She called Anastasia Maria Catherine and prayed for a quarter of an hour. As such
she was your little bluebird of happiness. Beautiful little phrases, saying how much
she loved either you or me. And saying the Lamb of God. I cuddled her, of course,
but cannot remember the murmurings of the Bluebird of Happiness because of the
Church Trial. She did six years Pope's Trial with me. I did another six months
afterwards for her with my mother. On Jan 20th I put her back in her cot after hearing
her first words – I had not taught her to talk – and went downstairs. It was midnight,

I went outside. There was one very bright star above the house.

It was on the pillow that she had her affair with either you or me.

For the rest she was sitting up when I woke. Difficult to see in the dark. I saw cosmetics

for five nights, and heard the prayers which like yourself were a miracle.

Please will you supply the missing prayers to the Pope? She said she was Mary.

I do not underestimate the importance of cosmetics. The light from her eyes echoes the blue flowers on her white counterpane. Will you make the case?

Mad and funny – seeing cosmetics for five nights. Mad and it involves me, my early childhood. I was almost there. I should have been there. It was just after I left Dad and Corinne in the house in Bath to be reunited with my mother and sisters and meet Frank in the new house at Waterloo Road. I only ever saw baby Amanda (Anastasia?) once, with her mother, when my sisters and I went to Bath for Christmas – a month before the events in the letter. She and Corinne both disappeared after that. The church trial seems to be the separation from my father. Corinne was from a Catholic background and divorce, difficult for anyone at the time, would have been more difficult for her in her mental state. And among it all, terribly sad, the six-month-old baby, a little bluebird of happiness.

I didn't talk about any of this with my father. None of us ever did – nothing from his personal life. My mother's vivid, difficult life was laid bare on the kitchen table at home, but of my father there was nothing. How he lived when we weren't there, most of the time, was kept from us. How my ex-stepmother and her daughter lived. We only knew Corinne was in a hospice in Kent. Did we still have a younger half-sister, Amanda? We weren't allowed to ask. Verboten.

It will be years until I ask my father just a little about Corinne, after she died. When I mentioned the flood of letters that came all those years ago, he sighed, said how dreadful it had been with her illness. 'I was besieged by those letters. I didn't know what to do about them. I couldn't reply to them, couldn't talk to her. I wasn't even allowed to contact her. The doctors said that anything to do with me would be too much.' I sympathized with him, saw how he had suffered too. But he hadn't suffered like Corinne. That had been wrong. The system was terribly wrong. No one should be shut up like that for the rest of their adult life on account of their mental problems.

'Fresh memory link, Lionel.'

'Fire away.' He leans back in his chair, closes his eyes.

'It's the blue flowers on the white counterpane like a newborn baby's eyes. I went to my father's flat in Chelsea with Lise. In November, 1972.'

It has flown in straight after reading Corinne's letter. We arrived in the evening at his tiny flat on the King's Road. Although the space was so small and crammed, Dad had created a marvellous oasis of calm. There was a white circular Habitat table under a spotlight, and in the centre a vase of cornflowers of the most intense blue. It was a wonder, a creation, the essence of cornflower blue, and he had made it out of next to nothing. We had supper at the Table with Cornflowers and then stayed the night, squeezed in on the floor among the kitchen cabinets. It was a great privilege to sleep there and the only time I ever stayed with my father in his London home.

'Some blue for your painting,' Lionel says. 'Cornflower blue and white. You can see blue all right, can't you?'

I see it again, the white circle of the table, the intense spots of blue at the centre, maybe just a bit off-centre.

'Let's think about this letter,' Lionel says, steepling his hands, eyes still closed.

27. Out of the tunnel

And it lightens. I lighten as though with the growing light of spring, if that's not too fanciful. Corinne's letters, Mum's breakdowns, a sister's problems, ruptured family at a young age, rebuilt family – they all recede. The big black cloud seems to float away of its own accord. Has Lionel helped? He must have. How much? I could easily say it was all down to Lionel – and how he listened, how transforming all that was – but I feel something else is at work here too, something cyclical, of nature. My depression has run its course again. Like one of those meteorological lows that blow in from the Atlantic and cover Cornwall, the south-west peninsula, sometimes the whole country, it has lifted and gone. *Suddenly I feel I have no problems at all. Thinking about other people, the rest of my family in particular, my self loses its enormous stature.*

Thom has moved out of Falmouth to the big house of Penjerrick, sharing a ground-floor flat with Canadian photography student Kent. It's another of those amazing old Cornish houses, in grounds sloping down to a wooded creek. What a wonderful place it is, a sprawling tropical garden, with specimen trees gone wild and huge ferns. There are great camellia and magnolia trees. The sodden hairy black trunks with great stretching fronds are tree ferns, he tells me. I love their primeval feel. Thom's room looks out on all this.

I rarely see him in college – he has a base in Sculpture somewhere, but his real base is in his head. He's a different kind of mentor for me, he feeds me ideas. These ideas are so at odds with what I do: pictures to hang on house walls, or public building walls, a school, office, library – if I'm good enough. I've come to think of him now as something of a Mark Wallinger, a maverick artist, a true original.

'Built-in obsolescence,' says Thom. 'In the future every machine will be built with an especially short lifespan. A car will last five years, a wristwatch two years. It has to be like this in the capitalist system, otherwise there won't be enough work for people. We have to keep on making things regardless of whether we need them. Repairs?' he laughs. 'In ten years time you won't be able to get anything repaired.'

I take Victor Papanek's book *Design for the Real World* away with me.

We look at Buckminster Fuller's geodesic domes. First written about in the forties, the potential of domes has hardly begun to be realised. Yet they are the buildings of the future, Thom believes. It will take almost until the millenium for one great realisation to appear in Cornwall with the building of the Eden Project in St Austell's china clay pits.

Lyall Watson. It's curious that Thom should be so impressed by him. Everyone's talking about this quasi-scientist, heebie-jeebie and paranormal expert, Lyall Watson, who has brought the weird and unexplained in nature to the public in his book *Supernature*. Thom seems happy to go along with his ideas, even with Uri Geller's spoon-bending, which seems to me just wacky. The aspect of *Supernature* that appeals to me, as the title suggests, is that nature is still full of unknowns, infinitely so, magic if you like.

Thom is interested in Chris Welsby's time-lapse nature films. And Wilk has also been asking me about them up in Photography. During the darkness of my winter, while collecting my Stowell's medal in London, I went along with Clare and Richard to a showing of Welsby films at the Slade. They were like a new species of nature film, about the earth, the planet, very physically about our planet. Most memorable was one called *Seven Days*, an early time-lapse film made in the Welsh hills, in which the camera on a tripod and equatorial mount (used to track stars) tracked the sun for a week, pointing at it when it was behind clouds and at its own shadow when it came out; as well as the fascinating weather systems, days racing past, condensed into a couple of minutes, the shadow of the tripod showed the rotating earth.

Chris is invited down to show his films and he makes the long trek from London on the train. A country boy, he calls himself, though I've only ever seen him in the thick of it in London, at the Slade, in Clare's flat. After his talk I take him for a drink in the Summerhill. We walk along Atlantic Terrace admiring the panoramic views over the harbour. I enjoy showing him round my Falmouth patch. I'm definitely on the up.

'26 good hours' is scribbled in my diary. I go to the pub on a Friday night 'heightened and intense after a day's painting', and Sarindar, the Asian girl from Canada, is there. She's full of laughter all evening and makes me laugh. After closing time we find ourselves still together, teetering down Jacob's Ladder. We end up at Desdemona's, a rather crummy little nightclub in the High Street, then go back to her flat above the launderette and sit up all night drinking tea. Love is in the air. It's come round again after all this time. Suddenly everything under the sun is there to talked about with Sarindar. My diary mentions me pontificating about art – and I see that Black Dog really does seem to have taken a back seat now.

Sarindar and I stay up until dawn. Now our ambition is to see the sunrise. We wait, drink more tea. At first light we walk in Arwenack Gardens and pick the municipal flowers – bluebells and tiny white jonquils, gorgeously scented. Ravenously hungry, we go back to Swanpool Street for a big fried breakfast. Then she leaves and I fall asleep, a deep sleep, not waking until afternoon with the barking dogs. Thom's at the door and Mrs Birch is apologizing for my still being in bed. They – Thom and Sarindar – call again. She hasn't been to bed at all, her eyes are smudged with tiredness. But she's still laughing. She's so lovely when she laughs with her strong teeth. Thom takes us for a drive to the north coast, to Portreath, where we walk on the pale yellow sand, climb on the sharp mussel-thick blue-black rocks. A sea mist rolls in and we go to warm up in the beach café with a pot of tea. We get back to Falmouth in the evening, and at last she leaves to go to bed. No, she doesn't come back with me. I'd like to say she came to my house then ... Actually, I'm just going in when I meet Kent and others and we pile into his car to go back to Thom's at Penjerrick for spaghetti and wine. Then we drive back into town to the Summerhill. I hang around, still drinking, hoping she might turn up.

At closing time I go on to Desdemona's and end up in the kitchen talking to Colin Smith again until the early hours – he's become one of those people I only ever meet with a glass in my hand. He tells me about the German artist, Karl Weschke, who has been his mentor. Karl lives out at Cape Cornwall on the Penwith peninsula. Expressionist, lover of ancient myths of Cornwall, he too paints in dark colours. He doesn't like the 'Cornish light' of the St Ives painters – he closes the curtains and paints by a 60-watt bulb, says Colin. Like Ray, who admires him too, Karl pits himself against nature in order to paint it. Later, he will say some things about his family life which strike a chord with me: how he put family and children first, before the art – that was partly why he painted at night by the 60-watt bulb. He seemed a hard man, thuggish, when I saw him in the studios. But reading about his harsh early life in Germany puts him and his paintings in a different light.

I finally return to my room, sit on the warm paraffin heater and think of Sarindar. Suddenly everything is happening again.

I'm back at the Launderette as soon as I can, hanging around her, mothlike. It must have been suffocating for her. At last I reach out and put a hand on her shoulder. And she freezes. My arm steals around her, she remains rigid; her body tells me no. 'Sorry,' she says, she doesn't want sex right now. Not with me or with anyone. Can I understand that? I can't really. It's a sock in the chin for the old male pride. Sarindar doesn't fancy me, plain and simple. So I stop chasing round to Desdemona's for a while.

Part Three: From Alba to Marrakesh

28. The circus is in town

Camels are browsing on the heath at Pendennis Point. There's an elephant in the gorse. Simon and I make our way to where the French circus trailers are parked around the edge of a field. We've come direct from the Labour Exchange for a day's work: putting up the circus. We got the job, were handed the owner's name and told to get up there straightaway. We don't know what we'll be doing, just that we'll be paid cash for the day. The boss strokes his chin and sets us to work. It hardly seems possible we can put up this huge marquee in time for tonight's performance.

Everyone mucks in, from bare-chested fire-eater/strongman to young children. The great centre pole is winched to vertical. A dozen ropes that radiate from the top are fitted to side poles, angled outwards to make the circle. With shouts and curses, knocks and bruises, it gradually takes shape. The enormously heavy canvas is dragged over the top and pinned down with guy ropes. It's ferociously hard work.

At some stage we troop over to a caravan for a break, and the talk, inevitably, is about running away to join the circus. 'C'est dur, c'est dur …' they say, but Simon, all Lindsay Kemp and Ballet Rambert, is up for it – he's acrobat, clown and small strongman rolled into one. One of the performers is a member of the embryonic Cornish Footsbarn Theatre and I can see Simon joining them.

Then the inside of the marquee. We create the wooden sections of the ring, erect the banks of stands, the plank seating. Everything is dragged, pushed, humped into place. The curtains, the lights, the sawdust. It seems to go on for ever.

A long day, yet how simple: the bottom line to have the tent up for the show, whatever the chaos and exhaustion behind scenes. At last it's done – half an hour before the start – and everyone disappears to dress. Simon and I hang around waiting to get paid, we wonder whether to stay for the show. But the job isn't over yet. The boss comes up, says he's sorry they're short-staffed, and we are needed. He gives us greasy grey shop coats and tells us to get in the ring! The music strikes up and we're leading the ponies round. It's just a few turns of the ring but we have to stay until the end. Then we have to fight for our money. Finally we get paid – the grand sum of £2 for a fourteen-hour day. The boss shrugs. Circus life is hard, there's no money. Simon and I crawl to the pub before closing time with our earnings and spend the lot.

Then I get together with Kate. One evening after the pub we end up in the Swanpool Street kitchen. We have some toast and I realise she isn't leaving. She's waiting for me. It's like first girl and boy – it always is: first time is the first time. I finally reach out for her hand across the table and her hand stays there, turns, clasps mine. It's decided. We stand and kiss in the kitchen. We go to bed. Her body is small, very white. She gyrates her hips, clasps me powerfully inside. It is short and very sweet. She leaves in the morning and there's a gap of a day or two.

I call on her in her shared student house on the hill. Her room is upstairs. The curtains are drawn, the room dark on a blazing afternoon – of course she knew I was coming, we have arranged it in the loose-easy way of then: see you Saturday afternoon. We embrace and now she holds me fiercely. I want to say that we went to bed and made passionate love all through that hot Saturday afternoon, but we don't. She holds me so fiercely, is so needy, I retreat. I'm really alarmed by her intensity. I don't want this at all. I want fucks, lots of them, with everyone. In truth I'd be happiest, I think, spending a night with every girl in the whole art school. But I don't want this urgent clinging. I'm not into deep relationships.

I back off in the darkened room, delay things. Suggest a walk along the cliffs as we half arranged. She's happy with that. We walk out of town and take the cliff path to Pennance Point and beyond – a long way. We clamber down a rocky slope and lie in the heather. We small-talk, talk about everything but. We're out in the open, it's so public. I think we have a swim, or we talk about having a swim. And that's about all we do. We don't achieve the intimacy of the night before at all. She goes back to her room and I go back to mine. Quietly, it's over before it has even begun.

Soon afterwards I see her in the pub on another arm, and outrageously, I'm jealous of this bearded black-haired Polish guy from the foundation year. That thing we do, mainly men: I don't want you but I don't want you to have someone else. I wasn't given enough time, I dithered. I was scared, yes, by her passion. I was shocked more than scared. I'd never experienced such intensity and need. And I have lost her.

Kate will lock herself away in that intense-looking relationship for some time, a year or more. I'm always aware of her and the flashing tooth of her partner. What was so daft, I think now, I realised even then, was that she wanted sexual experience from someone who knew, and I wasn't able to come up with it. Why wasn't I? I'd had enough experience. Why did I back off when she needed me? I kick and cuss myself.

I go after more experience and find Hester. It's the night of *Jaws*. Seeing *Jaws* in a packed cinema in Falmouth in summer is quite an event. The resort town of Amity Island becomes our Cornish seaside town, beaches packed to the gills with swimmers. The winding-up of tension with the invisible shark around all our legs as we wade through the murky water is unbearable. Waves of fear pulse through the stalls when the great monster at last breaks surface. The screams! I come out shocked, drained, yet somehow exhilarated, and go for a beer in a nearby pub. I find a group of students and sit with them. Suddenly I'm a rogue Great White myself, talking to this girl Hester, whom I hardly know, asking if she'll come back with me. We go to bed. It doesn't go so well, or rather it goes strangely. She remains uncomfortable, needs constantly to be touched 'there'. She holds my finger on her clitoris for the duration and doesn't appear to enjoy it at all. We don't discuss it afterwards. In the morning we are sheepish, and next time we meet in college, almost strangers. She was after some experience I wasn't able to provide.

Now Lizzie from Birkenhead. I know Lizzie from drawing trips, where she's rowdy and disorganised, and from her noisy table in the pub. She's a Scouser and she turns on the Scouse talk for me in bed. It's very funny. We lark about naked on the sheets on a warm summer night. She's voluptuous, heavy-bodied. I'm a skinny waif. We have just one night together, and that's fine. That's what she wanted too. She isn't expecting me back, and nor is she freaked out when we meet in the pub next time. There is that odd moment of a past intimacy but we know we've moved on as we should.

The Complementary Studies project is out of the way. In the end I abandoned my 'grand design' house in the dry valley at Colham and did a rather tame project on Gyllyngvase Beach. I needed to take a panoramic photograph of the beach, a 1976 version of a fabulous detailed panorama from the 1920s. Wilk showed me how. He gave me slow 32 ASA film and a tripod, and told me to use it on a bright day. Cloudy-bright was best. The result: a packed summer holiday beach, everything in focus, evenly detailed, just what I wanted. I added my oystercatcher photos and some close-ups of sea anemones in rock pools, together with maps and graphs for my visual essay on the town beach – all very A level History-cum-Geography and unsatisfactory.

Next I make a 16mm film. I have a go at filmmaking à la Chris. Since his visit in the spring I've come up with a number of ideas for my own little nature-inspired films:
Clouds racing across a small patch of sky, looking up through group of buildings or trees – in real time but would seem unreal, speeded up.
Huge sun and moon rising (or setting) just above horizon. The way the moon shrinks as it climbs in the sky.
The harbour with boats coming and going.
Penryn estuary tides rising and falling. Both these in time lapse.
Starlings on the art school lawn. Coming and going, groups, singles, moving across.
Pennance Point, my favourite local landscape – trees, shoulder of land, sea and clouds, ever changing. Fixed camera. Time lapse?
Constantly changing Cornish weather: Mon 26 January warm and sunny; Tues strong west wind, rainy, grey; Wed colder, north wind to gale force, sun and showers.

I settle on a film about time and tides in the harbour: how the small basin of the harbour drains at low tide and fills at high, how it completely empties to mud and almost brims over at spring tides. The dozens of boats sink onto the mud, then rise bobbing to the top. Wilk makes me sketch out a plan. Using time-lapse I will film a single spring tide from high to low to high over twelve hours. I check the moons in the calendar and settle the date for 24 June. The waterfront is too busy. A safe, undisturbed place to set up the camera would be on the roof of a concrete rain shelter overlooking the water. Up there I could just get on, click on the frames at the required rate with a little help. It works: the day is sunny; the little harbour drains and refills; the light changes from morning to afternoon to dusk. My helpers Lizzie, Carol and Wilk climb the ladder to the shelter roof and share the clicking on every couple of seconds for 12 hours. No sound. I don't think to put in sound.

For a time I become interested in the narrative film project that Carol, a curly-haired girl from Liverpool, and Lizzie's friend, is working on. Actually I am more interested in Carol. But *Harbour* remains my one small film. 16mm, colour, silent, 6 minutes. I show it at my degree show.

I start another harbour painting nearby. This one I'll do outside on the spot. I find a tucked away private car park overlooking the sea and set up my easel – bring the big easel down from my room, don't bother with any permissions. The weather is good, days of uninterrupted sun and wind. When the wind gets up in the afternoon I tie the easel to the rails. I work stripped to the waist, tanning myself, enjoying the salt and sweat of it. A few tourists come to watch – which I hate. 'Are you painting that?' 'Mm.' 'Look, he's painting that.' But I'm out of sight of the main drag, the endlessly drifting crowds, and am mostly left alone. To paint *an immensity of deep blue water, from lapping reflections below to horizon at the very top of the canvas, a few bright dots of orange buoys, white sails.* That's the idea. I spend a week on it, leaving the easel tied to the railings overnight, and finish it. In my degree show, the caretaker will tell me *Blue Harbour* is his favourite picture in all the shows: just the deep blue sea. I'm so pleased that I give it to him.

Build up slowly from thin to thick. To maintain freshness everything must be kept loose as long as possible. When leaving the picture it should have fluidity, giving it endless possibilities for the next time. A gradual tightening up, until at the end it's tight and solid, but at the same time loose and alive.

Then I do some pictures for the money. I knock up a dozen watercolours of the harbour to pay for my summer holiday in France. Like Schwitters in the Lake District after the war, painting scenes to sell to tourists, his real work put away. These I do in the open, board on knee, now *wanting* people to stop and watch. Which they do in droves – and I still hate it. 'Look, he's painting that.' 'Is he?' 'Yes, see the boat over there ...' In the evenings I have a job washing up at a café run by the enterprising Daisy May, who employs a bevy of attractive waitresses. She puts my watercolours up on the walls. They are pleasing enough objects and I wonder why they don't sell more. Are they 'too good' for tourist taste? Or not good enough?

I send a postcard to Mum in Tone Vale. She has gone in for a massive nine weeks this time.

> I hope very much you are getting better. Please try and do lots of drawing etc. You should sit on the bench in the Beatrix Potter orchard and do some – this is an order … I'm well and working flat out at watercolours to flog to the tourists. It's been hot & sunny every day. I get up early and look around the harbour when it's at its best, cool and fresh with lots of bustle and fishy smells, the sea still.

I stay washing up at Daisy May's among the waitresses and earn my holiday money that way – I think Daisy buys one watercolour in the end, or I give her one. Then I'm off to France with Simon.

31. Alba, Colham and Notting Hill

We take the train down to Montelimar in July, heading for Simon's parents' holiday house in Alba-la-Roche. We hitch the last part – walk to the edge of town on a baking hot afternoon and stop at a roadside bar for an icy beer.

Diary: *Simon's house in the middle of a medieval village. Tiny streets, massive stone walls, arches, alleyways. A 100-foot volcanic plug, La Roche, core of extinct volcano, in the garden. We walked up to town in the evening, heard the tinkling calls of bee-eaters.*

On the second night, a very hot night, I have a Falmouth, Colham and, I suppose, Alba dream.

> Leafy swanking with his guitar to an art school audience, dressed in white, *my* white nylon shirt. Everyone waiting for Pasters to appear and play drums. Eventually he arrived and now *he* was wearing my white shirt. They played but the atmosphere was awkward, embarrassed. Then silence. Pasters, feeling dreadful, said, 'How're you doing, Froy? We can always rely on you …' Silence. Everyone listening to me. I couldn't reply, no word would come out. Then A. was on the stage commanding the audience's attention, but we gradually moved to Colham on the lawn while still in the student common room. A., loud, preachy, was annoying me. We began to argue – I could speak clearly – calling each other fools. Now fully at Colham, night, I was in the ditch beside the barn. I heard Simon sobbing in the darkness and ignored it, pretended not to hear. He was calling me desperately. I finally called out to him to come and he appeared next to me in the ditch. I reached out to comfort him, stop him crying, and we were in a bed. He was asking me to love him. Please, just do it to me, I won't do it back. I was

writhing about but he was stronger and I knew he would win. He was going to rape me. I woke feeling sick.

I was aware of Simon sleeping badly in the next room, sighing, getting up to turn on the light. We'd had a furious argument in the evening after a lot of wine. Now I have to go through his room to reach the loo. The dream is still vivid. I can still feel him gripping me, wanting my comfort. I walk past him to the bathroom.

I've brought small primed boards to continue with my outdoor work of the summer. The days pass. We paint our pictures among the vineyards of Alba, drink wine in the evening. Don't argue again. The painting isn't up to much but I'm having a good holiday. There are delicious cool pools in the rivers for swimming.

15 July. Cycled to river pool beyond St Thome – pool full of hungry roach; also a small snake, sandy with blotchy back, triangular head. Collected juniper berries. Black redstart.

19 July. Day washed out with torrential rain. Walked along the river. Golden Orioles calling. Swallowtails.

20 July. Cycled to Sceautres, 8 km uphill. Wild valley. Climbed the great black basalt rock (another plug) which had a Madonna on top. Drew up there in the hot sun and wind. Alpine swift. Shrike swooping by road. Bee-eaters fly over Alba every evening. Black redstarts common.

29 July. Civilized comfort back in Alba after 3-day hitching marathon. First we went to Vallon Pont-D'Arc in Ardêche gorge, camped beside river under natural limestone bridge. Tried to catch massive roach at dusk, lost line and fell in. Continued down Gorge, hitching seul. Walked 4 hours before a lift. Great views from wooded mountains to twisting green of river far below. Arrived Avignon evening after long day's hitch on baking hot roads. Simon already there. Got drunk. Silly exploits – acrobatics in the square, climbing lampposts – before getting out of town and sleeping by road. Severe hangover in morning, only a loaf of bread between us. On to La Fontaine de Vaucluse by bus, 14 francs on fare leaving us 16.50 each. F de V a marvellous blue pool at foot of mountains, source of Sorgue. Cousteau dived 500 feet there and didn't reach the bottom. Purest water I've ever seen. Fast and crystal clear over green weed. Then the road back, penniless, cracking head and nausea (hitching is such fun). Walked 10 km. Finally picked up by some students who brought me right back to Alba. Luxury of waking up here, a cup of coffee, wipes out all the discomforts.

It's still hot in England. Hotter than ever. As hot as France. It has turned into the scorching summer of 1976. I leave Simon eating his father's gnocchi in Richmond and go to Colham to join the summer holiday there – we are back in the house at last after the long let. The valley is brown and yellow, grass burnt, river the lowest I've seen it, shrivelled to a trickle, weedy and smelly. The kingfisher and heron are still around. Harvest is already finished; the ploughed field on Truckle Hill, where I stop as ever to look for a Roman coin, is dust.

I go up to London with Clare to get some work. Turn up at the Labour Exchange, ask for a holiday job which needs no qualifications, and get one: general labouring in an Oriental and Persian carpet warehouse in Wembley. While waiting for the job to start, I return to Colham for a few days.

12 August. Yesterday a lovely shower of rain followed by a wonderful evening of misty tones. Today dry and sunny again, sun slowly moving across a sky of heavy haze, the air absolutely still. Snipe by the river above the weir, a first for Colham.

14 August. Beautiful sunny day, fresh and clear with a breeze. Walk upriver with Catherine, seeing at least 4 kingfishers, a dipper, grey wagtails, marsh tit and willow warbler. 3 hawks circling and frisking above valley: smaller than buzzard, broad wings with fingers, long square tail, brown underneath with lighter unmarked wings. [Sparrowhawks?] Back to the grime after idyllic 4 days and a successful yellow landscape of the heron tree and valley.

That 'successful yellow landscape' was big.

I took oil paints and a board left over from France up the valley to my favourite Colham view of the heron tree and beyond: sweep of the wood, hint of the meandering river, glimpse of the village at the head of the valley. I sat in the yellow thistly field through two hot hazy afternoons. Painted quickly, bringing the board back to prop up in the outhouse. Which was where Dad spotted it. When I returned on the second evening he said he liked the picture very much and would like to buy it. We looked at it and he wafted his hand over various parts, saying how good they were, particularly the fading to distance in the trees. Well, was it luck again? My palette was more discerning than before; these were 'my colours', the dried grass and turning trees, the light blue sky; autumn and winter are my best months for landscape. Anyway, he bought it for £25. Marvellous.

I spend the end of the summer working in London, sleeping on the floor at Clare and Richard's. Film-maker Chris is still up in the attic with his girlfriends; there's loud opera and much rumbling of floorboards. Richard is 'on the bins' for the vacation, working as a dustman in Willesden. I have my job in the carpet warehouse in Wembley, which mostly involves delving through great piles of Asian and Oriental carpets to fulfill orders. It's hot, dusty work.

One sultry evening after clocking out, I happily accompany Richard to a nearby pub beside the canal. We drink ESB, the strongest beer they have. Pints vanish into empty stomachs and we float pleasantly away into books, films and world philosophies. Richard is at Chelsea doing painting but turning towards photography. He's keen to talk about his photography ideas, the square format pictures he has been taking with his Rolleiflex at Colham this summer. He's also already drinking too much and the job on the bins doesn't help – his day starts at 6 and is ferociously hard until 9 or 10, when the round is finished. Then, the day done, they repair to the pub for the rest of the morning. There are special pubs for thirsty dustmen open at this time of day. Richard gets great biceps and a tan this summer but also adds to his drink habit.

I find time to see some Howard Hodgkin paintings at the Kasmin Gallery. I love them, how they are about 'the emotion of colour'; their brash confidence, the broad brushstrokes laid on, overflowing the frame; how they build up over many layers over time, yet are so fresh in the end.

It's Notting Hill Carnival weekend, just a short walk from the flat in Kensal Rise. We go down to Ladbroke Grove early in the day, Clare, Richard and I, are absorbed into the bright crowd, the red, yellow and green of the Rasta flag, the cobwebby dreadlocks, the noise. The steel bands at close hand, those rippling shimmering sounds that can be got from a tin drum, are astonishing. It's very loud. Everyone yelling, singing, screaming. Close-pressed bodies dancing. The air filled with meaty smoke. Ganja smoke further spicing the air. There's danger in the air too, the pushing, pickpocketing, an edge of violence. We follow the floats through the narrow streets, under the Westway flyover, with our cans of beer.

We walk back to the flat to rest our ears and have a break. Make a detour to look at 'King Faisal's' house, which is famously being squatted. Rasta flags hang from the fine Georgian windows. I think I'll see try and live there when college is over and I come to live in London – and I do call back a year later, climb the steps and knock on the grand front door. A head pokes out of a first-floor window and I make my enquiry: 'Any rooms going?' An Aussie voice tells me to piss off.

Then in the evening we stroll back down to the carnival – into a riot. Everything has changed, though you can't see it. The air is electric now. We walk right into it: a rush of air, breath of fear. We're suddenly inside a stampede of fleeing people. No option but to go with them, retreat from whatever it is, try to work our way towards the edge. Then we see it: an advancing tide of police, bobbies with their helmets, armed with truncheons and dustbin lids! With bin lids, traffic signs, cones, and whatever else they can pick up in a hurry. No tear gas, no riot gear as we know it. A bunch of bobbies off the beat, unprepared.

They draw up in a line, several deep, make a block at the crossroads and just stand there. The crowds jeer and boo from all sides. They pelt the Fuzz with missiles. There's no response from the police but a gradual thickening of numbers; they hold their ground, rained on by the missiles. Reinforcements continue to arrive, filling up from behind, and remain there, stuck in the middle of the road, sitting targets. They are bombarded with rubbish. Smoke from overturned cars blazes in the dusk. It's extraordinary, frightening, exhilarating. The police just stand there getting hit. You feel anything could happen, and quickly, the situation get right out of control.

We get out, thread our way through the crowd still growing to taunt these sitting ducks of police. Behind them, no traffic, the Grove closed. We walk back to the flat.

The papers next day report 350 police injured (and only 150 revellers), 36 buildings looted, 35 police cars damaged. Apparently, the cause of this 'race riot', the first of a fresh spate of riots at the carnival in coming years, was the rough-handed arrest of a pickpocket during the afternoon, and a young police officer being hit by a thrown brick when colleagues came to help him, which started a series of fights along Portobello Road. But the police were caught totally off-guard, outnumbered, outgunned by the number of people and their outrage. We read what's in the papers and our sympathy lies with the rioters. The Notting Hill Carnival becomes famous worldwide after this riot in the summer of 1976. A minute of ITN news film has been saved and can be found on YouTube. Joe Strummer, soon to be of The Clash, was there and will write the song 'White Riot'. What we saw was certainly a black riot but the origin of the Carnival in 1959 had been a response to mob attacks by white Teddy Boys on the black residents of Notting Hill.

30. In a caravan

September, my third year at Falmouth, last year at art school. I buy a scooter from dirty Clem 'the mechanic' in Sculpture for £25 – as though with my earnings from the Colham valley painting. It's a heavy machine, sprayed matt black all over, but a good runner, says Clem. I get a provisional licence and chunter round the high-hedged Cornish lanes. Freedom! *Zen and the Art of Motorcycle Maintenance* come to life. I make my little 'chautauquas' as I chug up and down the lanes. I find a dead seabird on the verge, a little auk, such an uncommon and special bird, which the driver who hit it probably has no idea about. I spy some tall stately mushrooms in a field, identify them as parasol mushrooms with the help of Richard Mabey's *Food for Free* and take them back to cook. I find *Psylocybe* too (not mentioned by Mabey), magic mushrooms with their distinctive little nipple, and eat one, and another. Nothing happens – there's no trip. Pete in Reading told a fabulous tale about running down some hillside high as a kite on magic mushrooms. I know I haven't had enough, I'd probably need to eat twenty of these, but my caution comes to the fore, that same caution that has kept me away from LSD.

Ken Kesey's 'Acid test': if you haven't tripped, you haven't been there. I do feel I've missed out, haven't quite been far enough along this particular road. Pete took it. Lots of Reading people have. Simon seems to have spent his sixth form crossing the road from his school to the University of Reading campus to trip out under the trees. I've read Carlos Castaneda's *The Teachings of Don Juan: A Yaqui Way of Knowledge* like everyone else, and imagined all sorts of trips with the peyote cactus in faraway Mexico. Actually, with me it's partly to do with opportunity – no one has ever passed me an acid tab at a party, on a picnic in the woods, on top of a mountain. Would I have taken it then? Not sure. Could have been persuaded. Ever since my bad dope experience in Mark's flat in Camberwell, though, I've been wary of the down side – at heart I feel I'm probably the sort to go off their rocker with a bad trip. I'm a Syd Barrett, a Peter Green, one of those who really shouldn't be taking that stuff. And this last year in Lionel's chair has hardly put paid to it. But instincts aside, a small source of regret remains: if I could guarantee my mood, a summer's day out in the sunshine with friends, then of course I'm up for a good trip. But I never do. I never drop acid.

Riding around the lanes, visiting Ponsanooth Wood, I find a small caravan to let. It's on a farm above the wood, high up with panoramic views east over Cornwall to the china clay peaks in the distance. I take it at once. The farmers say I'm the first art student they've had and they want me to do a painting of their house for my first month's rent. Now art students don't do picturesque farmhouses … but then again, when the money's this good … I choose a spot above the farm, a smallish canvas, and try to make something acceptable. The greens, the bright green fields, soon start to turn funny – aren't greens difficult – but I hold them down, I think. My landlords seem pleased enough with their picture for the mantelpiece.

The caravan stands on its own patch of grass above a lane. There's water from a hosepipe from a mains tap. Calor gas for the cooker and lights. No electricity and an Elsan toilet. The double bed pulls down from the wall. It's a joy. I park my black motorbike outside the door and know I can make this place home.

I cook a simple meal, wash it up in a little water, chuck the bowl of water into the hedge, rinse the crocks down at the tap. Vegetable peelings go on the compost heap, I fetch my pint of milk from the farm. At dusk, I carefully light the gas mantles without touching them with the match. They flare up, burn brightly white – I've damaged a mantle, poked it with the match, and the fragile gossamer curls apart as it burns; but I can replace it, you can still get such things from a hardware store. I close the little curtains. The caravan echoes to my footsteps, it creaks and rocks in the wind. I study *Food for Free* for what I can get from the land: nettles for an intense peppery soup, sea lettuce from the rockpools of Gyllyngvase as a slimy vegetable.

Now I bike into college, park in the car park below the studios. The gap in the hedge falls out of use. I still have to walk up the hill to sign in but all these fears seem to have vanished. I've stopped seeing Lionel as a patient.

I start a new studio painting – of the white studio screens. A white painting. I've anticipated Robert Ryman's White on White show at the Whitechapel Gallery by a year! Kasimir Malevich's *White on White* of 1918 has long anticipated me! But my painting has nothing to do with these abstract concepts, it again tries to be about light. Another bash at what's in front of me. I make my biggest stretcher yet and this time size the canvas only. The natural cotton duck will be my background. So, white screens, light falling on grubby white studio screens. Strange as it may seem, I'm after a very subtle painting of whites here. The open doorway in the corner of the room has a blue purple glow to it, which I render as a thin translucent layer – and it looks good.

Diane notices it. She comes ooh-by-gumming through the studios. 'Ooh, luv that purple bit! Full of light and space, in't it. Wonderful.' Diana speaks intensely in her Lancashire brogue, eyes bulging, and with such warm enthusiasm it can enter your work. Ah, the happy accident, the occasional magic of painting. I love that glowing purple patch too and not knowing how to repeat it I hold on to it.

Diane has only recently arrived from Preston and, I've noticed, has got together with Dick. She is a 'hyper-realist' painter, does marvellously real interiors, infinitely careful and painstaking, which she gets into the Royal Academy shows. She vividly describes the painting of a bedroom she's doing in Dick's cottage in Mevagissey and I want to see it. An opportunity arises when they are collecting some things from the cottage to bring to Dick's new house in Falmouth, and I'm invited along with them to view the painting. It's upstairs in the bedroom on the easel, in progress, and very large in the small low-ceilinged room. It's of the bedroom, mainly the double bed with an intense red cover. There's a cranefly flying over the bed in the picture and its model is a real one, a dead cranefly, suspended on a thread from the ceiling and stirring in the draught – the only sign of life in the painting. To me this picture is an astonishing rendering of reality, a realism I long for but colourwise will certainly never achieve. Diane says the sunlight through the window is only like that for a few minutes a day, and then only for a few days; after that you'd have to wait until next year. Diane Ibbotson's paintings of the places I knew around Falmouth are viewable online now.

I keep on thinly painting the paint-splattered screens in the studio. Someone leans their bicyle against a screen and I put it in. They take the bicycle away and I leave it part-painted – half a bicycle. It keeps me going for six weeks, this painting of screens in whites and greys, the red bike, the purple doorway, and in the end seems to peter out. I can't see what else to do with it, so I leave it. At my degree show I will sell it for the grand sum of £100 – to a couple, I note, who famously scour the shows for investment potential. Another sale!

The white screens painting is finished and I don't know what to do. Suddenly there's a new and different crisis of confidence in my work. I join the group of dissenters in the canteen – how different the canteen, the change in six months; how everything can always change – and listen to the same argument that painting is elitist and useless, and craft is what's wanted. Learn how to make something useful as well as beautiful, says Johnnie. Pasters is inclined to agree, except what he really wants is to fool about in a band. Thom wholeheartedly agrees about crafts being superior to paintings to hang on the wall, but he doesn't object to uselessness. Thinking of Thom, I'm reminded now of John Baldessari's 'I will not make any more boring art' of 1971, and of the Arte Povera movement: *Artist's Shit* by Piero Manzoni. Thom tells me with relish how Manzoni made 90 cans of it – 'contents 30gr net, freshly preserved, produced and tinned in May 1961'. I hear Thom chuckling. Is there really shit in that sealed can? Is it his? Is it a cow's? Bullshit! Does it matter whose shit it is anyway? Who's going to open it to find out? Who's going to open it when it costs all that money? The original price was the equivalent weight in gold, $37 at the time. The highest price paid to date, for tin 83 at Sotheby's in 2008, is £97,250. Manzoni then goes on to make *Artist's Breath* – balloons filled with his exhalations.

This all leads me down the basement steps at Woodside one Monday morning into Pottery. I've turned up to do a week's work, to learn how to make a pot. A bit late in the day, you might say, but there it is. The tutor is keen and helpful – I appreciate how seriously he takes this third year who needs a rest from painting. We'll make a good set of pots together. So I'm taken through the basics of clay again, not for a sculpture this time but for something useful: I 'wedge' the clay (slice it with a cheesewire, mix up the slabs for homogeneity), 'knock up' the clay (whack and knead it to get rid of air bubbles). I sit at the wheel, the amazing, impossible wheel, and gradually the spinning ball of clay begins to behave, some recognisable shape appears. I take to it, the physicality of it, the kneading, squishing and shaping; the magic of having a form rise up in my hands on the wheel, only to have it collapse in a shapeless mass, and straightaway building it up again. There are technical things to learn about each clay you use, its properties, elasticity. How far will it go? How high and thin can one make the walls of a pot?

The Monday–Friday element to the work is good too. Discipline, regularity, putting in the hours; 9 to 5 if you like. All of which also apply to painting. Though not, I think, with the way I've been battling with it, an infinity, driving yourself on with the work, ten, twelve, fifteen hours of the day or night, not stopping, really, because there is no end. You don't know where the end is when you are young, you must just push on and on and on. But you *can* learn to pace yourself with painting. Do your four hours a morning, carry over to the next day and build it up.

With the pottery, I just make a start. I work with a simple bowl shape on the wheel, always trying to get it thinner and lighter, lose that thick base. I pursue a wide rice-bowl shape, after the exquisite thin conical forms I've seen in Chinese and Japanese porcelain. I look at Bernard Leach – doesn't everyone, especially in Cornwall – and am drawn to a raku tea ceremony bowl. Ugly, squat thing! Misshapen black bowl that's had 'an accident' in the kiln and thus become special, revered. Beauty in ugliness. The accident that makes the special tea bowl is Zen.

I stay down in Pottery for two months, through the end of the autumn term and into the winter term. I learn to use the wheel and throw bowls, mugs and jugs. I attend to the biscuit firing, glazes, and the final firing. I want the natural colour of a glaze. Which is most appropriate for the local Cornish clays? I don't want pattern – only the true beauty of the form. There's so much to learn by trial and error. The plan becomes to make a 'set', which I do after a fashion. My jug comes out best, well-thrown, bulbous, with a good lip (you make the lip on a jug with a light touch of a finger) and a handle that works, fits the grip (you just wet and stick it on). And my bowls are just beginning to approach the desired rice-bowl shape. I use tin glazes in white speckly finish, in brown, in oatmeal. It's so easy to spoil the pouring and swilling of the glaze. All doubts and hesitations will show up in the firing. You must be swift and sure.

Then it's done. The experiment is over and I go back to painting. Pottery wasn't my vocation. But the set of crockery will go into my degree show as finished and useful objects. I've gained from the experience, appreciated the workmanlike practice, craftsmanship, great skill that goes into making a pot. Now I must get my skates on. I have a whole lot to do before the degree shows only a few months away.

Babs makes me up for the third Christmas disco. Dark-curled Babs has come to the art school now. She has Simon's old room in one of the college buildings. And I've had this great offer from her to get my face made up. I ride in from the caravan and change into my borrowed dress. Whom did I borrow it from, I wonder – Babs? It's silky and diaphanous. There's a wide straw hat with a ribbon too. Do I wear tights?

Babs sits me down in a chair and looks me over.

'Mm, good high cheekbones.'

'My mother's.'

'Women would kill for them. An actor's,' she says, rubbing in the foundation, accenting with colour.

I'm proud: Helen the actress in me; Mum's high cheekbones. I find I have some sense of wonder at my face as Babs applies the highlights, the shadow, the mascara, the lipstick. I moue my lips in the mirror, put the hat back on. And though I hardly remember it, I'd say she dresses as a man that night, goes in coat and tails with a topper. It's an androgynous time.

At the disco I drink a lot of beer as usual. I drink more than usual. The Christmas disco dance is an extreme event, we have to let our hair down somewhere in Cornwall and this is it. Tony has also come in a nice frock, without a beard. He's shaved off his long bushy beard for the occasion and is unrecognizable. I lose Babs to Thom, dance with my tutor Diane instead. We have a 'disco' friendship, Di and I. We find each other on the dance floor. *Voulez-vous couchez avec moi ce soir.* We don't sleep together, but twirling with abandon, breathless between dances, I remember, we compare our favourite Russian authors. She's reading Dostoevsky and loving him, recommends *The Brothers Karamazov*. I recommend *The Idiot*, whose hapless hero at the mercy of his epilepsy I identify with. On the dance floor there are a couple of 'cats down from London' (prospective students). I dance with Diane to impress them, glass in hand, twirling my long silky skirts. I'm telling them Falmouth has this wild scene that can compete with anything the capital has to offer. I know Diane enjoys the ambiguity of dancing with a guy in drag.

31. Ponsanooth

There's another party, in Redruth, at Wilk's new place with his new girlfriend. I ride over there on my bike. It's a bare boards and booze party, rather *outré* for Falmouth. And remarkable for the fact that Wilk has left his wife and family to set up with first-year student Susan. I'm not aware of any illegality of tutor/student relationhips at this time, I don't think anyone at Falmouth is, and they are quite open about it. I meet Susan's friend, Melanie, a dark-haired girl with milky skin, and we make it that night on the boards where we've crashed out. Next morning she comes back with me to the caravan. First girlfriend in my Ponsanooth home. I remember Ray calling round and expressing his relief that at last I have a companion in my lonely eyrie. It's fine with Melanie, easy going, love in the folding bed we swing down and leave down. She arrives one day to put me into a project she's doing in the wood. This becomes our most memorable event together. She dresses me in a grey cloak, tousles my hair, makes me up (again) and photographs me down in the woods as some fantasy Tolkien figure, an elf or hobbit. Recently, thirty-five years later, I was walking round the lake at the university campus here in Reading and saw a similar scene. This time it was a man photographing a woman in 'elvish' costume among the falling autumn leaves.

Melanie and I last for a month, then fizzle out.

My sister Catherine comes to visit me at the caravan; I cook her a rice pudding with orange juice because there isn't any milk, she remembers. I show her the marvellous woods and we hitch to the pub in the evening to meet my friends. I'm glad she has come to see me; our delicate yet strong spider-silk bond still holds us together. Catherine doesn't know what she wants to do yet – maybe it's art too, she hints. But she knows she's going to

London, has to get away from home. She's following Lise and De Gruyter's advice in that too. I think she's happier, slowly finding her feet.

I'm enjoying the physicality of living in a caravan in winter. Don't mind the water tap business, the loo with its reeking blue chemical flush, lasting the gas until I must hoik another cylinder into place. It's all part of being self-contained. I have my own small space in the world to look after.

Nights at the Summerhill resume, on my bike. One night, tanked up on beer, I come off the bike in the narrow lane by the caravan and fetch up in the ditch. Next, I'm giving Tamsin, a girl I hardly know, a lift back from the pub to her houseboat on the river at Penryn. We hurtle down the new open stretch of road on the outskirts of Falmouth as I always do – it's probably hardly 30 mph on that ancient 50cc machine – and the police stop me at the bottom of the hill. For carrying a postillion-rider without a crash helmet. They ask if I've been drinking and I say just a pint, and they let it go at that. I suppose because they already have me for the one offence, but it seems good of them not to breathalyse me as well. Eventually I'm fined £15 with two points on my licence. This is a substantial amount and I appeal to Granny Betty for help, which she gives. My granny pays the fine, for which I am eternally grateful. Tamsin feels guilty about the whole business. I laugh it off, insouciant and chivalrous, not blaming her at all, but she says she'll type my thesis to make it up to me.

Ray has bought a house, near Redruth and Camborne, the most industrial part of West Cornwall. He is also, suddenly, married and they're expecting a baby. I drive over to meet Geraldine, see Ray in the new family home. It's defiantly unpicturesque, set in a busy landscape of smallholdings and ruined tin mines, and it seems to me all he needs do is set up his easel in the garden, facing any direction, and paint exactly as he always has done. Yes, it's all completely amazing, the new Ray keeps echoing, as we sit in his big impractical house and drink tea, listen to his beloved Sibelius, look at the scruffy patches of moorland landscape beyond his granite-walled garden. But he's as keen as ever on drawing trips. Even keener. I haven't lost the Ray I know.

I start a marathon session of work in the caravan. It will be my last work and I think my best. It's the penultimate term, and whatever my misgivings about art versus craft, I'm now working hard on the art side.

On a warm sunny morning, one of those winter days stolen from spring that Cornwall surprises you with, I do my largest pencil drawing yet: the panoramic view from the caravan doorstep. I use a hard H pencil, so have to really work at the paper to get the marks to even show palely. It's the very opposite of my smeared charcoal, and has a light spaciousness. Diary: *In a spring landscape of racing clouds and sun, it's the alternation of light and shadow that is important. There's no need to follow it – it will return to what it was just as you change it. The pattern is what it's about.* Then it snows and I dash out to paint the evanescent snow, the brilliant fields in sunshine with strong blue shadows of tree and hedge. Seize snow or it will be gone, and by the end of the morning it has.

But mostly, now, I work from inside the caravan. I read *An Essay on Landscape Painting* by Kuo Hsi (11th century):

'Unless I dwell in peace and sit in leisure, with windows cleaned, the desk dusted, incense burning, and ten thousand worries drowned and subdued, I am not able to get at the mood and meaning of beautiful lines, think excellent thoughts, imagine the subtle feelings described in them. The same thing is true of painting. It is not easy to grasp its meaning. When I am responsive and at one with my surroundings and have achieved perfect co-ordination of mind and hand, then I start to paint freely and expertly, as the proper standard of art demands.'

Diary: *The more space that surrounds an object, the smaller it appears. The moon shrinks as it rises, the farm and stables diminish as I approach the caravan window.*

I become obsessed with the view through the main caravan window: farmhouse tucked under the hill, whitewashed walls. Put a jam jar of primroses inside the window on the table just in front of me – on the picture surface again. I work at my subject in pencil on paper and oil on board, make repeated versions, simplifying everything down to a few minimal elements. Distilling. It's abstracting itself – I'm on to something. The pencil marks are dark and soft again, made with the softest 6B enough of that faint scratchy H). Then I discover graphite dust, which I use with a finger. With graphite you can build the forms by denseness of tone alone. There are Seurat drawings like this, fuzzy-edged, simplified, elemental. Thinking of Morandi, I try to do the same in colour, simply: primroses in front of a hedge, a wild daffodil against rainy glass. I stick to my reduced palette, looking for subtlety, the infinite almost imperceptible variations of tones that can be made. I feel it's getting somewhere, but I leave off too soon, I know I do. Or later I know it. Colour gets me by the throat again. I abandon the primrose yellow and grey green, the fierce sulphur of the daffodil and rain grey. I push the graphite drawings further than the paintings but I don't push any of them hard and long enough. In the end there has always been that lack of killer instinct in me. Not killer, wrong word, I just mean lack of self-belief. I will take these things into college, put them into my degree show but know they could be better if I kept on pushing to the limit.

I'm also writing my thesis Abstraction and Empathy in the caravan, by gaslight in the evenings. It aims to illustrate

W. Worringer's thesis *Abstraction and Empathy* (1907) through Mondrian's journey to abstraction from his first naturalistic painting of trees to the rigid abstraction of Neo-plasticism – so far so good – and then attempts to tie in Frank's pure abstraction and my father's abstract landscape painting. Interestingly for me, Mondrian disliked green. He was all city: red, yellow, blue, black, white. He never used green in his abstract work; in his last great *Broadway Boogie-Woogie*, a riot of colour, there's no green. Frank doesn't use green either, but red, blue and mauve, and Payne's grey. Whereas my father is very green in his Wiltshire valley, whatever the level of abstraction. His kind of abstraction, I conclude, is empathetic with nature. I suppose I should be with Mondrian and Frank, but I like green. Greens, greys and earth browns are my colours. In a way, in retrospect, I share my father's love of landscape. Even if I can't tell a green double-decker from a red one.

32. Stuff of dreams

I move back into town, to Dick and Diane's basement in Stratton Place. They've been instrumental in getting me here, bringing me back from the wilds. It's easy here. I can concentrate on my degree show. I'm by the water again, further upriver towards the village of Penryn and Tamsin's houseboat. This part of the harbour is filled with small craft, which rest on the estuary mud at low tide, float off again at high water. Waking in the morning, there's the rattle of masts and rigging in the wind, incessant cackling of gulls.

Tom Cross lives along the terrace. He has come down to Falmouth like Ray. Last seen at the time of my collapse in Reading four years ago, he's my new professor. He learns that I'm a few doors away and invites me round for supper. Tom is bearded now, burly, altogether larger and more confident. His wife Pat cooks a delicious meal with a starter and dessert, which I never have. There's some conversation about our exits from Reading. But what I mainly remember is the grand wood-burning stove, the 'Pither', a stainless steel cylinder parked somehow in the middle of the stripped-pine floor and pumping out heat despite the warmth of the evening.

Wilk was also a neighbour on this terrace. 'Was', of course, because he's now shacked up with his new girlfriend in Redruth. His wife and family still live in the fine family house along the waterfront. It brings home to me the loss and tearing apart of divorce. I suppose Wilk, in love, can't see it yet.

And a new painter, Philip Sutton, is on the terrace. He has appeared at the college to teach and, I remember, joins a drawing trip with Ray – that's two tutors to four or five students. Philip does his rapid paintings. He brings along half a dozen tiny canvases and finishes them all in the day. He paints thinly in oil. Brightly. Gaudily. Colour is everything, he says, the joy, the liberation, the explosion of colour. His aim is to complete a landscape in a couple of minutes with just a few brushstrokes. Most of the time is spent preparing, building up to the moment. Then the doing. Zen stuff. If it works it works, if not, wipe it off and start again. Of course he produces a lot of paintings this way, he laughs, so it's better if they're small. He has a twinkle in his eye, Philip. He is small and lithe, exercises a lot, runs miles every day. He's also quite famous: looking round his house, there are scores of bright canvases of all sizes, maybe finished, maybe drying so he can continue with them, maybe on their way up to galleries or coming back from them. There are portraits and figures as well as these new Cornish landscapes. Most of all there are flowers, and I'm reminded of my mother's love of flower paintings.

After the exhilarating day with Philip Sutton, Ray takes a few of us for our long promised trip to Carnyorth on North Penrith. We drive through St Ives. In truth this iconic town hasn't meant much while I've been at Falmouth. St Ives painting is regarded as old hat and we're rather dismissive it, while the place itself is just another tourist trap. The artist Patrick Heron, another colourist, still works from his hilltop home above the town, but he doesn't visit Falmouth in my time. We pass his Eagle's Nest studio. We pass Lower Tregerthan in the old mining village of Zennor, where D.H. Lawrence wrote *Women in Love*; it's also where Peter Redgrove met Penelope Shuttle. Our hostel on the clifftop is a little further on.

I don't get much work done. I play table tennis with David Bratby (father an artist like mine, more famous than mine) and follow tortuous paths down to the rocky shore with the Bearded Wonder, who still wears no shoes. We climb on the moors to see the standing stones and dolmens, marvellous Men-an-Tol and Lanyon Quoit. Apparently Bruce Lacey and his wife have been up there recently, dancing around the stones, re-enacting and inventing their ancient pagan rituals. I watch birds rather than paint: spectacular ravens in the wind, auks on the rocks; I look for corn buntings, becoming rare, and the elusive peregrine I've still not seen in the wild; I imagine finding the Cornish chough, which is feared extinct now – would I be able to see its scarlet legs and bill? One afternoon we walk along the cliffs to see Rose Hilton. It's not long since Roger Hilton died and for Ray this visit is partly in homage. Hilton drank himself to an early grave, and as he did so painted some extraordinarily bold and free works which I don't yet appreciate – they seem very careless and messy. It will take me a number of years to come to appreciate this vivid painter. Rose is charming and kind, and we sit in her kitchen above the wildness of Cape Cornwall (where Colin's friend Karl Weschke also lives) and drink mugs of tea. She hasn't begun to paint in her own right yet – it will be some time after the death of her flamboyant husband before she again becomes a painter in her own right.

On Sunday nights my landlords make love in the room above my head. It's their routine. I hear them going at it through the ceiling. Seems they do it to get a good night's sleep for Monday.

My double bed takes up half of the basement and I spend time lying on it during the day. There's a stone wall just outside the window I get to know; a narrow strip of lawn, the sky. Yes, I'm lonely staring at a stone wall, and I'm feeling small. Someone said that while we sit in our armchairs (or in my case the bed) we're in fact turning a gigantic somersault once every 24 hours, and revolving at a speed of 700 miles an hour, and orbiting the sun at 18 miles a second, and travelling in the direction of Vega, together with the rest of our solar system, at a speed of 12 miles a second, and gyrating round the centre of the Milky Way at 170 miles a second.

Running upstairs to the ground-floor bathroom one day, I faint. I could so easily have fallen back down the stairs, cracked my head on the tile floor, I think, but I'm fine, I just carry on. It was an odd little aberration which hasn't happened since. But the sinking in my mind is not. It reappears in time for my degree show in a few weeks time, reappears *because of it.* I don't carry on painting and drawing up to the last minute, as many do. No, instead, I concentrate on completing my pottery, getting it glazed, finished and photographed for the show. I get my thesis finished and hand it over to Tamsin for typing. She has kept her word, her atonement, she calls it, for her part in the motorbike incident, for allowing herself to be driven home without a crash helmet.

While I'm kicking my heels, not painting, Dick gives me the name of a potter who lives on a distant creek of the Fal. I make a trip to her remote studio. Find a warm welcome and wealth of paper-thin, translucent, oriental-shaped pieces in fine white porcelain. It seems a fine life she lives there, surrounded by her work, endlessly creating. It seems she knows exactly what she wants. For years I think the woman I met alone among her pots in those woods was the famous Lucy Rie.

Oh the sinking feeling. I put off seeing Lionel again, resist starting all that up again. It isn't so bad, I tell myself, not if I keep busy. I wonder if it has something to do with the time of year. Mum gets her 'July feelings'. She gets depressed in the summer. Is this to be my inheritance too?

'Beaky', a wild bottle-nosed dolphin, has been frequenting the harbour – he's become curious about several small boats and taken to following the Flushing ferry.

I'm fascinated with the sightings of the dolphin, this great ten-foot animal living in the harbour now, so trusting of humans. At least I am interested in Beaky. I keep a look out but never do catch a sight of him.

I'm still writing down my dreams in tiny script in my notebooks. I still don't date them, deliberately enter them at random so there will be no sequence 'as in life'. A girl called Vanessa in the foundation year has disturbingly entered my dreams. I continue to dream about both my homes

In a train compartment I disturb Kate and Vanessa naked, getting into bed together. Kate thinks I'm deliberately intruding.

In bed in the attic at Colham I wake and find Dad, a bit drunk, in a good mood sitting in an armchair. Clare and Catherine are there. He says he's invited Granny Helen and Tully for the rest of the weekend, they'll be flying over tomorrow. Catherine H and Francesca have gone away and Dad is trying to recreate the old family atmosphere.

Walking down Waterloo Road to our house, Chris Welsby is behind me. He has a beard and shaved upper lip. He says Clare's kitten died while we were away. I open a cardboard box to find a different kitten inside. He explains he has replaced it without telling her.

Walking up a steep diagonal path on a grassy hillside with my sisters and others. The path divides into two, one doubling back, the other going straight on. I go on ahead as I've never been there and the path leads to a beautiful wooded valley. I go back to get the others. Clare and Catherine have already taken the other path because they know where it goes. The others have gone back to the start of the fork. I try to explain what a good place I've found but Clare insists on keeping to the old path.

There's a dirty scrap of paper with something on it. It's the envelope from Clare's letter I threw away last evening.

Now with Tom Cross in his large studio. I show him

> the scrap of paper, no longer an envelope but a drawing by Catherine covered in mud. He rips it up and throws it down, carries on painting, says this is how it should be done. I attack his painting as he works, smear the paint with my fingers. We fight as he tries to protect his work, which becomes small, blueish, Victorian, like Frank's, and completely different from the other large abstracts in the room. I knock him out and put him into a bed, the bed at Colham which Dad tucked me into. People come to congratulate me and tell me the little mud-covered drawing is far better than any of these big pictures. I start on a large abstract painting of orange interlocked shapes like Tom's and think it's good.

I continue to write down my feelings too, in some attempt to keep on top of myself. I write about my inability to choose a shirt in a shop. I spend a lot of time writing now, and don't know where to put it. I've been holding off. When I finally give in and go to see Lionel, find myself pleasantly ensconced in his room again among the figurines and ceramics, the redolence of Freud and Jung, he suggests I write some more. He strokes his moustache. 'Mm, why don't you put the story of the shirt into the third person? Someone else is buying a shirt.' So I write it down for Lionel. I try to put everything in, not caring how it looks. Actually, I find my personal horror turns into a bit of a comedy. On paper it hardly seems to be about me at all.

THE SHIRT

> He needed a new shirt. A new one had to be bought. He had shirts of course but none of them were any good any more. Indeed the more he thought about the shirts he owned the worse they got: the old denim friend, now threadbare, frayed at the collar; the hairy khaki army one, which was ticklish and needed a vest worn under it and was too sticky for summer

anyway; the odd slinky purple one from the Champs Élysées which could never be worn.

This new shirt would lie somewhere between the drab khaki and the shimmering purple. It must be both somehow: ostentatious but not, bright yet dull. He looked around (there were no charity shops in the town then) and found a cheap place with a whole rail of cotton check shirts outside on the pavement. Handmade in India, good price. Were they too bright?

'Can I try this one? Actually these four? I'm not sure which colour …' The boy in the doorway with arms folded, on shoplifting watch, nodded and seemed to smirk.

Inside the cubicle, he liked the red and navy one but it was way too small. The red one fitted but it did make him look pale. The blue and white one was too contrasty. The other red and blue one had too much blue; it was a bit vivid and on the large side. The collars were large on all of them, he noticed. Didn't they make small collars any more? He tried on the four shirts again. Each had their pros and cons. He emerged from the cubicle at last and bought the first one, the small uncomfortable one, which was the best balance between showy and invisible, and hurried home.

In front of the mirror, it was clearly the wrong shirt. He could hardly move his shoulders. Still he hesitated, wasn't it also rather flattering, accentuating a lean look? If his face were a bit more tanned … Remembering this was the flattering mirror, he went to check in the bathroom, where he had fainted just the other day. Whether a mirror was flattering or not depended on the angle of light. When the light came from behind, he thought, his reflection was ugly. From the side, it was okay. The flattery level also changed through the day: worst in cool light of morning, best in mellow evening. Bad in the north light, where so many self-portraits were painted. He knew all this from doing his own self-portrait – it wasn't just from vainly staring at himself in the mirror.

It was still morning, but he was going to have to change the shirt.

He couldn't get back to the shop until the next day – which at least gave a chance that the smirking assistant might be different, making it less embarrassing to change an item he had already spent hours trying on the day before.

It was a radiant summer day, the harbour a millpool, reflections of the boats mirror doubles, but this all passed him by. He hurried to the shop and it was the same sales assistant.

This time he didn't ask. He took six or seven of the check shirts off the rail and went straight into a cubicle. Half an hour passed before he emerged and swiftly exchanged the 36" for a 40" in the version with more blue than red. Back home in front of the bathroom mirror *it was too big*. The collar was enormous. How could he ever wear this enormous flashy thing? But maybe in the bedroom mirror in the evening light, or in the strobe light of a disco ...?

Oh it went on for days – it's still going on. He couldn't take the shirt back again so he decided to remove the two ridiculous lapels, and then the top pockets, slicing them off with a razor and having to make repairs with needle and thread. He tried it on. Better. Okay under a jersey or jacket. Then you hardly noticed it.

He went out in it. Walked through the busy streets of the thronging seaside town and no one seemed to notice. He looked hard at all the people but they didn't look back at him. In the canteen queue at college no one mentioned the shout-aloud American cowboy shirt he was wearing. Were they blind? No, they weren't interested and why ever should they be?

‘How does that feel? Any better?’ says Lionel.

And we laugh. We have one of our belly-aching laughing sessions.

‘Where is it? I can’t see it. We can’t see if you’re wearing a shirt at all under your jersey,’ hoots Lionel.

Then he leans forward in his chair, cracking his fingers. ‘I know what you mean about that ticklish army one. Absolute nightmare. Tell me about that one.’

So we talk about ‘my time in the army’ in the CCF at school, how I hated it: from horrors of the Assault Course to the baking-hot quad on Friday afternoon parade. And our conversation turns back to the nightmare of public schools for a while. Of course so much has been written on the subject, right back to Dotheboys Hall. It’s the pain that sticks with me, still, when I read about public schools. George Orwell’s misery at school rang bells for me, as has Andrew Motion’s recent description of ‘the Tickler’ in his childhood memoir *In the Blood*.

Lionel doesn’t ask me about the purple shirt. It’s as though he’s saving the Champs Élysées for a later date, though there won’t be one. We never do get round to talking about that shirt.

I go to watch the harbour on a lovely evening, climb the hill above Swanpool Street to the top road by the Sea View pub, sit on a patch of grass there. Because I once saw her walk past here at this time. I smoke and look at the view and my thoughts revolve around Vanessa. Vanessa, this girl I know in my dreams but have hardly spoken a word to. If she comes by here I’ll ask her to stay and talk, go for a drink.

And suddenly there’s her voice. She’s passing a yard behind these railings. Talking to someone, an old man. I finally I turn round and catch a glimpse through the railings of the little figure disappearing round the corner. She’s wearing her starry T-shirt and jeans rolled to the knee. I stay where I am, apparently looking at the boats with renewed interest. Will she come back? Why would she return this way?

What to do? I stand up and dither. Go home? Go for a drink? Walk to the beach? It will be quiet on the beach at this time, beautiful in this light, and the water warm enough to swim. But who wants to go to the beach alone? I have to buck up. It's the end of term. She'll be going off for the summer. Indecision whirling, I go for some fish and chips, eat them slowly, walking along the top road, find I'm back where I was before. I sit on a bench in the sun, making the chips last. Watch the boats, the crowds of little Mirror dinghies with their pastel-coloured sails still out on Carrick Roads; there's heightened activity around the huge black-hulled oil tanker which at last looks as though it might be going to leave. A drink? Yes. The Sea View.

And there she is again, alone now, walking towards me, fifty yards away along the straight road. I can't reach the pub before we cross. There are no side roads or turnings. I almost turn and run, can feel my body twisting away from the encounter. The gap closes fast. Twenty yards. Fifteen. Ten. She smiles, but too early, too far away. She can't hold it. Five. My face contorts.

'Harrghro,' I grate in Martian. Her face clouds. I caused that. Now she's worried. Fear flashed across her face for a moment. At the point of passing she looks down. Then she's gone and I'm in the pub, steadying myself against the bar.

Frank's words echo. 'Whatever you do, John, don't try to drink yourself out of these moods. It's what your mother's been doing for years. It's how it starts.'

I drink. scribble on an envelope. Vanessa has gone. Twice in an evening. I scribble back, front, inside and out.

Then I'm outside her door. Number 11. I know the number. Ring the bell. No answer. She's out. How lucky she is out. Laugh. Go on, laugh.

Walking to the beach at sunset, trunks and towel under my

arm, I try to work it out again. What actually happened? *He* became paralysed. Powerless. At the crucial moment he couldn't act. Then all that was left to do was go and see her. Tell this person he didn't know all the things he thought about her – if only he could get out of this obsessive way of doing things. Just meet her, talk to her. This at least he must do. He's knocked on her door once. He has to try again. Maybe he doesn't even need to try, for this is bound to happen again. There'll be another of these non-meetings on the road. *You cannot change yourself. You will only do the same again. The only way to change is to recognise how you should change and then seek help*, I read somewhere. Learning comes from hang-ups, someone else said – when you are forced to sidestep, try another path, because the old way is no longer enough. Fate is trying to help me. I mustn't ignore it. A month ago when I passed Vanessa in the same place I felt the same. The feeling has been pushed to the back of my mind, but it hasn't gone away at all. Now it's telling me again.

Lionel is less impressed by my account of not meeting Vanessa. He's looking out of the window at the sunny morning, dreaming about something. When he's really listening he either stretches back in his armchair with his hands clasped loosely over his stomach, his eyes closed, or he leans right forward, teeth bared. He thinks I should just get on with it with Vanessa. Or not.

In the end I wrote to her. I put some of the above in a letter and posted it in her door. And she replied. Her letter reached me several months later: she was surprised … flattered … actually the feelings weren't altogether one-sided. She was back home in Ireland now but maybe we would meet again one day. And that was that.

'The Sex Pistols!' yells Lizzie in the Summerhill, where I'm drowning my sorrows. 'Punk, John! Punk is where's it's at!' The

Sex Pistols take a while to get through to me. I miss the media hullabaloo – I would have enjoyed their famous F-word moment on TV, one of the first on television, especially so shockingly early in the evening. (I don't watch TV at all, or even read the papers now. Art students don't.) Yes, the first punk I hear is just a tuneless racket to me. *They can't even play those guitars.* Punk won't reach me until next year in London. Then I'll come to like that anger, bitterness and contempt. Johnny Rotten's 'Anarchy in the UK'. I want to be punky too, wanna yell *I don't care.*

My thesis is ready. I collect it typed and bound from Tamsin's houseboat moored at Penryn and stay the night. I'm surprised when this happens – it wasn't part of any plan – but then I see how it was always on the cards. A night rocking on the river, water gently slapping the boat. She says I can stay again, any time I'm passing.

It's show time. Time to put up our degree shows. I emulsion my studio space brilliant white. When it comes to getting out all the passable stuff, I find I've done more than I thought. There's enough. The canvases need batten trims. I join the queue of painters in the workshop to mitre pine strips and tack them to the canvases. I borrow a set of large frames for my drawings. My pots, the equivocal 'not-fine-art' pots, go into the show on a small table of their own with a set of photographs. And the etchings of the Goonhilly Downs radio telescopes – pity I haven't done more. I fill the fresh white space with my three years of endeavours, and hey, what an enjoyable experience. Simon is on the other side of the partition – his work is much more homogeneous than mine: paintings and drawings from life. My work seems all over the place. I give *White Screens* top position on a screen by itself, arrange the others around it, and a group of the framed charcoal drawings. I'm most comfortable with these, and they do best, winning the Drawing Prize. sponsored by English China Clays at St Austell – I'll present them with the drawing of their clay pits.

In the cluster around the results notice board on Woodlands Avenue, there are tears from the girl who gets a Third. Clem the mechanic fails as he expected. Thom suffers the injustice of a 2:2, but it won't appear to affect him – I see him rise above it, visiting him in the autumn in London, his small rented room in Battersea, which he has ingeniously doubled in size by contructing a mezzanine double bed in the redundant space under the ceiling, while he considers his next step; I see on the internet that he's still a practising artist now. Simon gets a 2:1, a good painting result. I get the same – what a relief. I look again at the Firsts: Dave's surprise film loop installation of a waterfall descending a series of screens made in Ponsanooth Wood. Kate's simple, refined show of just three close-written foolscap volumes of maybe half a million words.

But enough of that. The degree show Dinner & Dance is coming up. There's also to be a staff/student cricket match, a college tradition, which I'm curiously looking forward to. The invitation card for the dance is a photo of me in cricket pads and prickly gloves, shirt off, crouched keenly over my bat. We were having a practice on the lawn; I was batting, relishing it, being part of a team, such a simple thing, when Kent popped up in front of me and took the picture. He got me to sign all the cards like a famous cricketer autographing his bat.

Is the Dinner coat and tails? I don't remember. It isn't in drag at any rate. There's a tall girl, olive-skinned with long brown hair down her back, a Joan Baez, waiting by the entrance. She asks if she can come in with me, she hasn't got a ticket. Eileen, the beautiful American girl who left last year, back on a visit. She has just come from Ireland, is passing through, on her travels. I've only ever *seen* her before and she wants to be my date. What fabulous luck. Eileen takes my arm.

Then I lose her due to the seating arrangements. She's at another table through the long meal, the shenanigans – old Hewlett reading his traditional Verse to the New Graduates – and I fear I won't see her again. The tables are cleared for the dancing, and here she is in front of me. 'Am I still your date?' And we're dancing, and now it's working, the chemistry. We dance with others, with everyone, but gravitate back to each other. There's the final conga round the canteen and she finds me again. It's suddenly the end and yes, she would like to come back with me. Jesus God, I asked and she agreed. How I lark about, play the fool on the walk home, down the 111 steps of Jacob's Ladder in the dark, until we come to the harbour.

She's with me and the harbour is beautiful, the boats are slowly swinging on the tide. The water laps, reflections ripple, inviting us in. 'Let's swim!' Yes, now, it's not so crazy, I dip here all the time. The harbour is none too clean but it's just a step away from home. I try to persuade her to join me for a midnight swim, still horsing about, playing the fool to win her, and she watches from among the drawn-up rowing boats on the shore, but won't be enticed into the dirty water.

'It's warm. Gorgeous.'

'Be careful! There'll be glass,' she calls.

She stands on the shore, on the slippery seaweedy low-tide beach, watching me, with me. She helps me step back ashore, gives me my clothes and shoes. We cross the road to the flat and to bed. She lies on top of me and stays there till morning. Then she's kissing me awake and leaving. She has already gone for the train.

Our night lasted for another twenty-four hours, in burning sun, in caressing wind, in sweat and perfume of roses. How my sight and hearing were dulled, how my touch and smell and taste were alive. How good to be loved so fiercely.

I still can't believe it. She straddled me, took me inside her. She lay on top of me, directed the proceedings. She rocked backwards and forwards, her breasts brushing my chest. I could hardly come, I'd drunk so much. I came badly. Wondered how much it mattered to her. Then it didn't matter any more. I felt the intense romance of her.

She left at 6 a.m. for the train.

A card arrived next day. A photograph of Alice Liddell with her long tresses: 'Here's someone for your painting.' She said six swans were flying under the bridge at Penryn as the train chugged up to Truro. It keeps me bathing in the afterglow.

The art school cricket match is a ramshackle affair. We've had our one practice on the college lawn, the staff haven't practised at all. The *Falmouth Packet* turns up to report on it, take a picture of the teams. I look the utter fool, pissed at the cricketers' tea. I don't know the outcome of the match. The *Packet* doesn't actually say in its brief article: 'They toiled not neither did they spin …' But important for me was Pasters' grilling and my gradual disclosure of how I got off with Eileen, or how she got off with me.

'Never! With the American beauty?' cries Pasters, the expert on American girls. 'Froy, you old goat!'

He couldn't have paid me a higher compliment.

Kate and I go for a walk to Swanpool Beach and argue. My praise for the writing she put in her show, for her boldness in submitting that, and only that, gets a jolt. Our conversation walking along the beach shows our true opposing natures. It's almost Hewlett versus Redgrove. Chemist v. alchemist. Paint only what's there or paint wherever your imagination takes you. We look at the waves. She says they are animals, creatures, aliens, shapes of anything. For me they are waves, part of the system of tides, the daily rise and fall, and the wonder in that. There's enough without turning them into sea monsters. But how boring, she cries. Can't we imagine what might be there, just under those waves, even if we don't fully believe it? What's wrong with a shoal of mackerel, I say, gannets diving after them right now, even as we speak? There might even be a Jaws out there, I quip. It's as though she's showing me how different she really is, that I've been mistaken all the time. That really we are chalk and cheese.

I remained half in love with Kate, with some phantom of her, for a long time. A year later I would write to her from London (she was still living in Falmouth) saying how things were generally okay with my life and that all I needed now was a wife. I was actually hardly conscious of the blatancy of my words and wondered why she took so long to reply. Eventually a reply came, chiding me for my sexism but apologizing too for her 'compulsive need to analyse everything' – it seemed to me she had left the door ajar. Then there was another letter, which I'd forgotten about but which fell out of my notebooks, from UEA in 1978 – so she did get on the famous writing course. It took up my earlier invitation to come and stay at the squat in Vauxhall. But now I wouldn't be there. Great plans had been made, suddenly, and I would have already left for Central America. So we didn't meet up, we never did. I have no idea what she's doing, where she is, who she is now. I can find no trace. I always felt she would become well-known as a writer and wonder if she might be using another name, married or otherwise.

There's a beach party at Mawnan Smith beyond Swanpool, an end-of-everything party. I walk there along the cliffs, past where Kate and I spent our fruitless afternoon. It's already dusk, a warm night, and people are swimming. The dance floor is outdoors under a roof without walls. There's no Eileen. Thom and Babs are still going strong. I see Kate. Then I see Lionel dancing cheek to cheek with Kate. I see his eyes are closed. He looks in heaven and it pierces me. Kate is with Lionel. I keep hunting round but there's no one for me tonight. Nothing for it but drunkenness, with Simon, probably, who hasn't had anyone for ages. It's dancing with myself. And at midnight there's skinny dipping for all in the sparking phosphorescent sea.

Wilk has come up with the idea of a trip to Morocco during the summer vacation – vacation for him, end of college for me. Driving there in the college bus. He's thinking about six weeks of travel which might cost so much a head. I jump at it. Decided. I'll get the money together and go. That's still the sum of me, really. Earn enough for the trip and go without any thought of what's to follow; return without a bean, *no direction, no home.* I'll live like this for years. Until I marry, until I have a child.

33. Falmouth dog days

I get a job decorating a flat above a new bistro on the High Street. Ten years on, I'll start earning my living decorating rooms, flats and houses – I have no idea I'll be doing that. The bistro owners are the couple who bought my *White Screens* painting. They have great faith in me as a decorator too. It's wonderful to have people with faith in you. The job I've been entrusted with is simply to smother all the ceilings and walls with woodchip paper to hide the crumbling plaster underneath. And it works in a way, it binds everything together. I'm more than content to do this basic practical work and get away from my little daytime nightmares of shirt buying and writing to a lost girl: work with a beginning and an end, for which I'll get paid. It all goes into the Morocco fund.

Dee turns up one day. Married. She and her new husband Stephen have been away from Reading since she graduated last year, living in Cheltenham, spending an icy winter on the dole in Nairn, and have come to look at the foundation course here for Stephen. He's up at the college now and she has tracked me to my basement.

She comes bouncing down the steps in her playful puppy mode. Finds me lying on the bed in the afternoon – yes, back there again, L. Cohen style, examining my navel, perhaps re-examining my night with Eileen, and watching a strange insect with very long antennae creep along on my wall. Dee stays an hour, bucks me up with her super-abundance of high spirits. How odd that she should be coming to live in Falmouth just as I leave. Passing ships. The next time I see her, eighteen months later, here in Cornwall, it will be to fix up our 'arrangement' for Cocos Island; she is newly divorced from Stephen and I have asked her to come and be my desert island partner for a year. We'll sleep together after a night out in Redruth with her new friend Wilk, and meet again in London two months later to board the Freddie Laker skytrain to Miami, destination an uninhabited island in the Pacific.

In my basement I read Lionel's novel *The Pantechnicon*, a nasty story about what might go on inside the walls of a large anonymous white van and pass unnoticed by an oblivious world – the rape of a young female hitchhiker. It takes place in the south of France, where I've done plenty of hitching, where I met the Parisian girl Sylvie hitching alone, where Clare was nearly attacked.

One day Lionel tells me of the sad squalid death of John Magoldrick.

'You've heard about John?' he murmurs. 'Poor John's killed himself.'

How shocking it is to hear this. Always. And it always seemed possible with him. Every time I saw him recently. I want to know how, and Lionel supplies the answer without my asking.

'He took a whole lot of aspirin in the end.'

A memory flies in of a boy at school, Melvin, who had similarly rebarbative parents with a regimented upbringing. Melvin overdosed on paracetemol just before his A levels. He took a hundred, they said, but he survived.

It's been two years since John Magoldrick came back. For the first six months, back at the art school again, doing that mad red man painting, he was specially looked after – excused signing in every morning, given a college room – but he couldn't manage it. He left the college and stayed on in Falmouth, on the dole, of no fixed abode; hung around at Lionel's, Pat's, Lionel's, Pat's, Vicky's van. He got up at 4 p.m. and stayed up all night. He haunted the studios in the evenings. He had bad spells and went into hospital, several times, came out looking better. Then deteriorated again. Last winter, after a long absence, he was at the Summerhill, haggard and wild. By the summer term he'd reached his nadir, an old man in his early twenties shuffling up and down the road, just outside the only place he knew but was now excluded from. I walked with him once to the beach, Conversation was difficult, he was remote. He told me he was sleeping in Vicky's van now, opposite the college gate. His last trip had been to Inverness, he said: he took the train all the way up there, someone found him and put him in hospital – I didn't know whether to believe him. He was put on the train back to Hertfordshire where his foster parents lived, found again and taken to hospital. In July, he was back in Falmouth.

'The boy had no parents, he hated his foster parents, and they had disowned him anyway.' Lionel looks bereft.

'You did all you could.'

'Yes.'

It feels like the end of college for me. I applied halfheartedly for postgraduate at the Slade, and quite rightly wasn't even asked for interview. I've held back from the Royal Academy, which is surely too academic for me, though Dick and Diane think I should give it a go. I wouldn't presume to try for the grand Royal College. No, I don't think I'm going on to post grad.

There's the sense of an ending at Colham too, though it will be another year before we actually leave. Clare and Richard have come down from London. I walk down the valley with Richard, photographing the river. He's interested in the reflections and the river bed, the tension between surfaces in the picture – he always talks about his interests and aims in his work. Unusually, in the days when serious photographs are still mostly done in black and white, he makes large square colour prints of his work. They are among the last pictures taken of Colham valley.

Next year we'll be out. We will lose the house we feel we've always had. The 14-year lease taken out in 1964, when I was eleven, which we believed would last forever, finally comes up. The landlord has decided he wants to live in the wonderful Colham house after all, and Dad has to move on.

Maybe we remove some of the furniture this summer, or my memory jumps on a year. Chris Welsby comes with a hire van to fill with furniture for Reading. The evening he arrives I take him for a walk along the river towards the village. He asks me how my time-lapse film of the harbour at Falmouth worked out. What will I do with it? I don't know. What do you do with one film? Chris says he keeps the masters of all his films in the bank, which is impressive if a little precious at the time, though doesn't seem over-cautious now. I show him my valley: the fallen willow which has carried on growing where it fell, the clay bank where the kingfisher nested one year and where water voles can usually be spotted, the stark dead elms dotted like bones through the woods. I ask him why he doesn't have a camera with him, and he says he never brings one the first time he visits a place: if a place needs pictures taken, you can go back and do it. We stare at the landscape, which I know so well and he doesn't, together – he with his filmmaker's eye, me with my painter's eye. We stop to consider the solitary heron oak and slope of the dark August woods behind, the meanders of the river, the distant village church tower – subject of my 'summer of 76' oil painting which my father so memorably bought. Chris says he'd worry about things ending up 'picture-skew' (picturesque) here; it must be a problem living in a place as chocolate-boxy as Castle Combe.

Then it's back to the house and packing up, Dad being organized, deploying his forces. The oak cupboard that takes up a wall of the sitting room and once contained all our children's games has already been dismantled. Stan, the technician from Reading Fine Art, came down especially to dismantle it over a weekend – like some nineteenth-century flatpack, 'all dowels, hardly a nail or screw'. Stan will reassemble it in the Reading house. My father has always got on with tradesmen, craftsmen, builders. He admires anyone with skilled hands: 'Painting is so much about the manual skills.' He treats them with high respect and they like him for that.

While writing this book I learnt that Lionel Miskin has died. A Day of Remembrance was held for him at his last home in Bovey Tracey, and judging by the website many people came. I had lost contact with him after he left Falmouth and went to live in Cyprus 'for his health'; he came back to his wife Pru and they settled in South Devon. I drove past that village several times not knowing he was there. I missed his funeral. Wished I had been there. And I imagine so did a great number of others he nurtured through his long teaching life – many survivors! I read the page on the Web and smiled. How he would have loved the advent of the 'world wide web' and its sticky name.

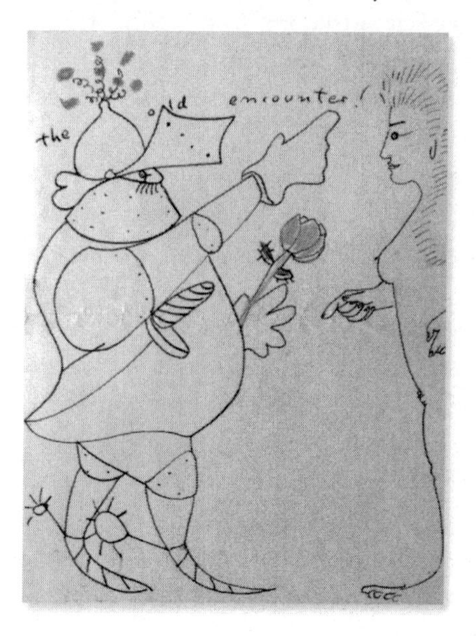

34. Marrakesh

We set off for Morocco in the art school bus, motoring up the A30 at a steady 56 mph. Wilk has been calculating how much less petrol we would consume if we stuck to fifty-six. It seems sensible to cut costs, though will make for slow going on the motorways of Europe. He does all the driving. I can't drive, though some of the group can. But Wilk is running this show and we are his student kids. We can take turns sitting in the front with him – Jack, the naughty one, can sit right at the back. Wilk is taking us all the way from Falmouth to Marrakesh and beyond, and he's bringing us back again. We'll go out into the desert as far as we can, to a sign in Zagora that points to the Sahara and says Timbuktu.

The white VW motors up the A30 at its appointed speed, across Bodmin Moor, the Tamar Bridge, with nine of us crammed in. Babs has come but not Thom. Not Simon. There are no couples among us and nor will any form during the trip. For some it's just the vacation and they will go back to Falmouth, carry on. For me art school is over, the work done. Where will the work all go? Where does it end up in the great post-art-school dispersal? Art is so bulky, and storage, especially of not such great art, is an ongoing problem. The *White Screens* painting was sold to the owners of the café; *Black Range*, that black thing, has gone to the staff room; *Blue Harbour* now belongs to the caretaker. The heavy, sand-encrusted *Swanpool Street Interior* 3 will go to Waterloo Road, where Frank will hoist it up on the wall and it remains to this day. *Interior* 2, looking through the windows into Mrs Birch's garden, Mum wanted; it will go up in her kitchen where she sits and dreams and never does any work. She's been quieter this summer, we think a bit better. *Window* with its funny greens has fortunately been left somewhere to moulder away. My father has the hot summer Colham landscape. Of the drawings, *China Clay Mountain* has gone to St Austell, and *Panorama* from the caravan was bought. The rest – the finished, exhibited drawings; the sketches, starts and stops – will fill two portfolios and go under my old childhood bed at home for a while, then accompany me from room to flat to squat to co-op to house, often a little out of sync. They will go under many beds, be looked at occasionally and reappraised, thinned out; some will be framed, some binned, others go back under the bed and move on. The pots will go to anyone who wants them – a couple of those bowls are still in use in our kitchen in Reading today; Clare has the jug that's a good pourer. *Harbour*, my 16mm film of the rise and fall of tides in Falmouth harbour, six silent minutes in its silver canister, will go into some college archive, and maybe it's still there.

We drive across France and Spain, cross from Algeciras, and land in clean North Africa. The complete lack of litter on the Moroccan shore is striking. I sketch distant Casablanca in watercolour. It's my last bit of painting for a while, until I'm asked to paint a sign next spring for Vauxhall City Farm, my new home in London. No one does any more artwork on the trip. We concentrate on improving our photographs with our in-bus tutor Wilk.

We head south into Morocco. I share a tent with Wilk and we're good mates. He talks about his young girlfriend back in Redruth, and is evidently still very close to her. He seems almost to be under her spell. I wonder why she hasn't come on the trip and he says it didn't appeal. I talk about losing girls. Kate. All my girlfriends since Lise.

'We lose lots of people, lose *the one* more than once. Find another one,' he says.

And the Black Dog in Falmouth. Which came first: losing the girl or getting depressed? You'd lose her if you got depressed;

you couldn't get her when you were.

'You'll survive. You'll get through,' he says as we lie side by side in the hot tent.

One night we are camping on the Atlantic coast, a barren red shore of thunderous surf, empty of people. The tents are pitched facing the sea to pick up any wind. There's always this fine balance between open flaps for ventilation and letting the mosquitoes in. The mosquitoes have got in. Just one mozzie inside is my nemesis. Through my thrashing about I'm aware that Wilk has been gone from the tent for some time. I hunker down in my sleeping-bag sheet, finally sleep, and wake with the sun already hot on the tent wall. I'm discovering my bites of the night when Wilk looks in, face all pink-polished and beaming. He's shaved off his beard.

'Try doing that with a blunt razor,' he mutters. 'Took me bloody hours.'

'But why?'

'Oh she wanted me to. I promised her.'

He surprises everyone at camp breakfast, grinning across his round boyish face. What a transformation of old man Wilk, the forty-year-old lecturer.

The rest of us guys are doing the opposite, we're growing our beards for the road. Mine is a first beard, and beginning to bristle up quite nicely. The guys, except Wilk, grow their beards, and the girls strip off in the growing heat. Or rather they do two things: bare themselves and swathe their bodies with thin gauzy cottons from the market. Something about these wafty clothes is as alluring as wearing nothing.

We head for the famous souk in Fez. But most of us don't get there, we've gone down with the trots. We bought these little homemade ice creams from a kiosk on the outskirts of the city ... The consequences were dire. I had such squits I couldn't leave camp for two days. Squatting thus in the desert is memorable –

the burning sun, squadrons of flies, jelly legs. Everywhere the smell. It seems that all humanity is continuously dumping its ordure outside the city walls. It all dries quickly, odours fade, the flies move on, but nature can only take care of so much of this at once, and our evacuations hardly helped the balance.

We drive on, dehydrated, weak. Acclimatizing. Make our camp under a clump of date palms by the road. There's no fencing, no visible division of the land (though remember that scene in *Lawrence of Arabia* when Omar Sharif comes riding through the mirage to claim his waterhole). No need for a tent, we bed down on the sand; wriggle in our sleeping bags into a comfortable hollow and look up at the incredible stars. How cold the desert gets at night. How rapidly it heats when the fireball bursts over the horizon. Photographing this parched land of rock and cairns of stones in the early morning light, the shadows still long, I sneak one of Babs, sinuous in her bikini.

In Marrakesh, we watch the snake-charmers with their baskets of cobras, argue about the Indian rope trick, bargain for leather bags and belts and chess sets in the souk, seem to acquire ever more of these flowing cotton clothes. I buy a jellabi – still expensive despite much bargaining – which I'll wear in the cold desert nights but never at home; it will hang around for years until I finally give it away. We join the communal tables in the main square after dark and eat with our fingers, dipping into the *tagine*, and we watch the *kif* smokers with their pipes on doorsteps.

We drive over the High Atlas on a fantastic road of hairpin bends. Clamour at Wilk to stop the bus for some hash. Jack buys a slab from a group of Berbers by the road, our stash for the rest of the trip, though Wilk will have nothing to do with it.

Now we come down into the great heat of the Sahara. The road follows a fast clear river that flows off the mountains to sink into the desert. We bathe in its wonderfully cool, mineral-thick water, where boys are swimming like fish, chasing fish and catching them in their bare hands. We stop at village standpipes for water, drench towels and wear them over our heads – they dry in minutes. Gone are the shorts and bikinis. We are now all swathed head to toe like Bedouin in our flowing robes. We stop to look at red-clay buildings, flat-roofed as it never rains, or with no roofs at all, no glass in the window holes. At one village the boys come round to taunt and jeer at us, throw stones at the bus. We flee. We drive as far as the famous Timbuktu sign, meet a German returning from the desert in his camper van, yelling 'Fifty degrees', which we translate into 120 Fahrenheit. Then we turn north and wind our way back towards the Mediterranean, and the heat hardly subsides. Camping in a breathless canyon, the rocks turn into grotesque animal forms with the cannabis. A camel train goes by in the moonlight. Really? Or was that a hallucination too? Still inside the canyon next day, we sit out the midday heat under a great awning strewn with rugs. The thermometer rises inexorably above a hundred, a panic-filling heat.

Now we're on our way home – to what, I don't know. Is my life half empty or half full? I know I'm not doing post-graduate. I'm going to live in London. Clare will be in London. There are all these new language schools. I could try teaching English as a Foreign Language to Italian students. We lie round the camp fire on our last evening in Morocco with the giggles and the munchies, trying to finish up the stash we can't take with us across the border. Everything is like a Happening or an Installation when you're stoned. I had one more big laugh with Lionel in his room in Falmouth, over Bruce Lacey, whom of course he adores. The thing about the Lacey way – his unending, challenging, controversial search for self-expression – is that it's fun, it doesn't hurt. As Lionel said, if you make an enormous jelly-shaped figure filled with fruit, and leave it in an East

London housing estate for the kids to dig in, where's the harm in that?

In my stoned state I'm 'with' Babs. Babs has, maddeningly, gone back to wearing an itsy-bitsy bikini to top up her tan ever since we left the desert.

'So why aren't *you* wearing your purple slinky shirt, that little number from the Champs Élysées?' she giggles.

'Because I'm wearing this one,' I say feeding the fire with sticks which crackle and pop, blaze quickly and subside to embers.

'What's so great about this one, then?'

'I'll tell you.'

I have on the Shirt, the cheap red and blue check shirt that caused such trouble only a couple of months ago, a shirt that now passes unnoticed. I tell the story of how I acquired it, this modest item, the terror and paranoia of being in that little shop in Falmouth. It all seems plausible enough, true and profound in the clouds of hashish smoke around our little fire.

I give the slinky purple shirt to Babs to try on. Of course it suits her. She's one of those women who seem to suit everything. 'Keep it,' I say. I want the mystique of Paris to hang in the air, even if it did actually come from a jumble sale in North-west London.

'While we're here. For one day. I wouldn't take it back to England,' she says and this seems extraordinarily funny.

Wilk doesn't join in with the giggling. He doesn't do drugs, not even an innocent bit of cannabis almost legally bought and smoked in Morocco. He's the outsider as we toke and bogart and pass round the joint. He waves it by, different, older, and I feel for him as the outsider. He was far more the outsider than I ever knew. He will drive us home and I will see him a few times in the Photography Department of the college, which I still feel fully entitled to use to print up my Morocco photographs.

Then the next time we meet in the autumn of 1981 he will be a woman. He'll have changed sex, really done it, gone the whole way. Old Wilk will have become Jill, with breasts and a vagina and an awkward way of holding a handbag. But that's for another story.

Babs doesn't keep the purple shirt but I do give her something. To express my adoration, probably misplaced and almost certainly unreciprocated, I get her a Michelin man. I steal her one on the way home. She was admiring them, these lorry mascots, white pneumatic creatures, all the way down through France – idly, I'm sure; she didn't actually *want* one. But I surprise her. Somewhere in central France, I spy a likely candidate on the cabin of a wrecked lorry. I cross the baking hot tarmac of this truck graveyard, climb on the cabin roof and wrench it off. It takes some doing. Hard plastic – hardly rippling pneumatic – well-bolted on, and up close also rather large. I bring my Michelin man back to the waiting bus and present him to an astonished Babs, my gift to her because I fancy her to bits. 'A souvenir of the trip. You said you wanted one.' It's a great big unyielding teddy. But she is pleased, flattered, and I am overjoyed. She'll keep him. She'll find a home for him in the cramped space of the bus. Michelin man doesn't win her for me, of course. When we reach England, she vanishes with him into a train station.

Two Rivers Press has been publishing in and about Reading
since 1994. Founded by the artist Peter Hay (1951–2003), the press
continues to delight readers, local and further afield, with its varied list
of individually designed, thought-provoking books.

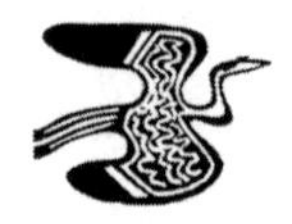